I0095267

LOW SODIUM COOKBOOK

A Yummy Low-sodium Breakfast and Brunch Cookbook for Effortless Meals

(Beginners Guide to Healthy Living on a Sodium-free Diet)

Nathaniel Shutt

Published by Alex Howard

© **Nathaniel Shutt**

All Rights Reserved

Low Sodium Cookbook: A Yummy Low-sodium Breakfast and Brunch Cookbook for Effortless Meals (Beginners Guide to Healthy Living on a Sodium-free Diet)

ISBN 978-1-990169-75-5

All rights reserved. No part of this guide may be reproduced in any form without permission in writing from the publisher except in the case of brief quotations embodied in critical articles or reviews.

Legal & Disclaimer

The information contained in this book is not designed to replace or take the place of any form of medicine or professional medical advice. The information in this book has been provided for educational and entertainment purposes only.

The information contained in this book has been compiled from sources deemed reliable, and it is accurate to the best of the Author's knowledge; however, the Author cannot guarantee its accuracy and validity and cannot be held liable for any errors or omissions. Changes are periodically made to this book. You must consult your doctor or get professional medical advice before using any of the suggested remedies, techniques, or information in this book.

Table of contents

Part 1

Introduction

Are you easily irritated by trivial things such as a skewed table in your room, or a tuft of unruly hair on someone else's head? Are you sometimes unable to focus on that class presentation you're working on? Do you often experience muscle weakness even during the early morning hours of the day? If you answered "Yes" to any of these questions, then you may have a high concentration of salt in your blood. You have eaten too much salt and the symptoms are manifesting in your body. Yes, these three are symptoms of hypernatremia, an increased sodium concentration in your system. One of the reasons is due to an increased salt intake. Aside from these manifestations of hypernatremia, there are various unhealthy conditions caused by excess salt in your body.

It's true that salt gives flavor to your food. Salt can turn a bland tasting dish into a succulent, edible cuisine. Salt, when used sparingly, is the magic wand for cooking savory foods. Yet, that table salt that we commonly label as "plain" really isn't plain at all. It's like a time-bomb waiting to explode in the hands of an irresponsible and ignorant person. Don't let this person be you. Read on to learn more why salt can be destructive to your health, and what to do so as to avoid its dangers.

Table salt is chemically composed of sodium and chloride. These two extracellular electrolytes or minerals are important in retaining the water-electrolyte balance of your body. Sodium has an active function, while chloride has a passive function. Sodium also has an essential role in the sodium-potassium pump that helps in maintaining balance or homeostasis in the body. Together with the rest of the electrolytes namely: potassium, calcium, magnesium, and inorganic phosphorus, they help in significant biochemical and physiologic functions to keep you fit and healthy.

The food that you eat is the major source of sodium and chloride. Maintaining the normal levels of sodium and chloride in the blood is critical for good health. A little less or a little more can spell death for you, so you have to be vigilant about what you eat. You must be aware what food contains sodium and chloride. Know that there are non-salty foods, which are rich in sodium chloride too. Being knowledgeable about all information regarding your table salt will assist you in preventing the health risks involved with its consumption. Since sodium has the active role between the two electrolytes, let's equate salt with sodium to facilitate this discussion.

Chapter 1: Health Risks Of High Salt Intake

Ingesting too much salt involves various health risks that could result in disaster for you. Before you generously sprinkle salt onto your food, make sure the salt in your body is still within the allowable salt concentration. According to the Dietary Guidelines set by the Nutrition Facts Panel of food labels, the daily salt requirement of the body is not more than 2,300 mg (milligrams) - that's about a teaspoon of salt.

For more susceptible individuals such as those who are middle-aged and older, persons with kidney and hormonal disorders (diabetes mellitus), or people with heart diseases, the American Heart Association recommends only 1,500 mg and below.

The lower the table salt intake - the better for you. This is because there are other food sources of salt. Salt is often used to preserve food because microorganisms cannot grow on excessively salty surroundings. Preserved foods such as processed meat, canned goods, and cured items are examples of sodium-rich foods. Even if you don't use table salt, there's already more than enough salt from your diet.

The increased concentration of more than 160 mmol/L (millimoles per liter) of serum sodium in your blood is termed hypernatremia. A decreased concentration of less than 120 mmol/L is called hyponatremia.

An elevated chloride concentration is termed hyperchloremia. Hyperchloremia has similar symptoms and causes like sodium because they're sparring partners. A concentration of more than 120 mmol/L leads to hyperchloremia, while a concentration of 90 and below is hypochloremia. Increased salt intake, without corresponding water intake, will cause hyperchloremia.

Hypernatremia and hyperchloremia increase your risk of acquiring the following diseases:

Hypertension

Salt increases blood pressure by increasing water or fluid retention in your body. This blood volume increase will prompt the heart to pump more forcibly to promote proper circulation. This will increase the blood pressure that circulates through your arteries causing hypertension. Hypertension can affect your major organs to cause several pathologic conditions.

The American Institutes of Health disclosed that hypertension can cause kidney failure by thickening and narrowing the walls of the kidneys causing less excretion of toxic waste substances. In this case, the waste products accumulate in your body and can only be removed through dialysis; a process where waste products are filtered from the blood to purify it.

Heart diseases

Hypertension, in turn, can lead to serious cardiac conditions such as weakened arteries, myocardial infarction (MI), Cerebrovascular Accident (CVA) and cardiac failure. These are lethal diseases that can lead to disability or death. MI is a condition where cardiac cells are compromised causing infarction or necrosis (tissue/cell death). CVA, in layman's term, is a stroke. Stroke happens when a clot forms in the blood vessels of the brain, or when the blood vessels in the brain burst and bleed. The excessive retention of water can also cause accumulation or edema in areas where it shouldn't be found.

Aneurysm

Aneurysm stems from hypertension. When your blood pressure remains elevated, the pressure of the blood can weaken your arteries causing them to bulge and eventually burst. This is called aneurysm. The rupture of the artery will cause internal hemorrhage too, which is fatal, under unmanageable circumstances. The bleeding can lead to blood loss, and then, finally, death.

Dementia and cognitive impairment

High blood pressure can also cause dementia and cognitive impairment due to the blockage or damage of the brain's arteries. With the existence of dementia and cognitive impairment, the risk of developing Alzheimer's disease is increased. Mental impairment and mental disturbances are equally common.

Impaired vision

Untreated hypertension can lead to impaired vision due to the bursting or bleeding of the blood vessels of the eyes. This could aggravate and cause permanent blindness. Before this happens, take preventive measures by lowering your blood pressure to save your eyes. Your eyes are your windows to the world; therefore you should take extra care of them.

Kidney diseases

Your kidneys are also affected. You have two, and therefore you could potentially survive with one dysfunctional kidney. However, you will overload one kidney in performing the functions of, supposedly, two kidneys. This could lead further to other serious conditions such as kidney failure or kidney shutdown.

The kidneys are the major excretory organs of your body. They are responsible in excreting acidic waste products of metabolism. When these toxic products are not eliminated properly, they will accumulate in your blood and poison you. Metabolic waste products are mostly acidic in nature. Their accumulation in your blood will considerably decrease your blood pH leading to acidosis, coma and then death.

A slight increase or decrease in the normal blood pH is risky. When it goes untreated, mortality always results. Nevertheless, the body's Central Nervous System (CNS) and Endocrine System (ES) will respond automatically to the imbalance. Once the pH disturbance is severe, the CNS and ES won't be able to achieve homeostasis in your body, unless diagnostic procedures and therapeutic treatment are initiated.

The kidneys are likewise involved with the hormones, namely renin, angiotensin, and erythropoietin. These are vital substances in normal blood pressure maintenance and red blood cell (RBC) production. Dysfunctional kidneys will lead to hormonal imbalances that will disrupt homeostasis.

In addition, there's also the danger of the formation of kidneys stones (nephrolithiasis) due to salt or crystal accumulation. Kidney stones can cause genitourinary tract system blockage that may require surgical intervention. In addition, kidney scarring and kidney failure can occur in the long run.

Water-electrolyte imbalance

Increased sodium concentration will prompt the body to take in more water to keep the balance. Too much water will give additional load for the organs to excrete. This balance is critical in sustaining the body's normal blood pH (alkalinity or acidity). The amount of salt should be in proportion with the amount of water in your body. Severe dehydration seen in diarrhea, profuse sweating, burns, and vomiting can cause hypernatremia, when you continue taking in salt, despite your water loss. On the other hand, hyponatremia occurs if you stop taking in salt; hydrate yourself properly; and sweat or urinate more often.

Worsening of Diabetes Mellitus

Increased salt concentration coupled with diabetes mellitus (DM) is a lethal combination leading to your early demise. DM destroys your organs, while accumulated salt would aggravate the destruction. Even though sugar and salt have different flavors, they both have harmful effects on your body. They destroy all your organs until nothing is left of them. You've got to monitor your consumption of these two harmful substances. It will be a sad story if you acquire an illness caused by these two because you were indifferent to the information provided here.

Osteoporosis

Osteoporosis is a disease where bones are brittle and weak because of insufficient calcium. Studies revealed that too much sodium can inhibit the absorption of calcium; this will consequently cause osteoporosis. Osteoporosis is one major cause of bone fractures, especially in the elderly. Love your bones and make them stronger and denser by reducing salt in your diet.

Blood gas imbalances

The water-electrolyte imbalance will likewise cause blood gas imbalance, in which the pH (alkalinity and acidity) of blood is disturbed. This will lead to either metabolic alkalosis or metabolic acidosis. Think of your body as a weighing scale that has to stay balanced at all times. If you tip that scale, there will be bad health repercussions.

Increased salt or sodium in your body is not only due to excessive salt intake. It can also be caused by conditions involving excessive water loss in proportion to sodium such as, profuse sweating, prolonged diarrhea, fever, diabetes insipidus and severe burns.

Chapter 2: Health Benefits Of Reducing Your Salt Consumption

Now that you know the unhealthy effects of too much salt intake, it's time for you to learn about the health benefits you can actually derive from reducing your salt ingestion. Too much of almost any substance that enters the body can potentially serve as a poison or be hazardous to your health. Salt is one such substance. Reducing your salt consumption is a major step in staying healthy, fit and trim.

Enhancement of excretion of waste products

Waste products are more easily excreted when the body is in a homeostatic state. When each substance is in its normal level, the physiologic functions proceed well, including your kidneys' excretory function. The proper disposal of your body's waste products will ascertain that the blood circulating in your blood vessels is clean and pure. It can be likened to a sewerage or drainage system where dirty water is discarded smoothly and efficiently because there are no blocked pipes or accumulated silt.

Prevention of cardiac, kidney, bone and hormonal disease

As discussed in the previous chapter, your heart, kidneys, bones and hormonal balance are affected in the presence of excess salt in your body. It follows then, that eating less salt will lessen your susceptibility and risk to the aforementioned diseases.

Your heart will be safe from heart attack, stroke and cardiac failure. Your kidneys will function reliably without the danger of kidney failure. The excretory system will run smoothly, and your bones will have ample calcium to develop properly. Your hormones will be in their appropriate concentrations to perform their tasks efficiently.

Why risk your vital organs just for that salty taste when you can safely use alternative food condiments? Treasure your organs; normally functioning organs are imperative to good health.

Maintenance of homeostasis

When water and sodium levels are maintained within normal values, homeostasis in the body is achieved. Homeostasis is critical in maintaining good health. The maintenance of the normal concentrations of all the substances in your blood helps all your systems in performing their physiologic functions, thereby, keeping you healthy. Chemistry books have established certain normal values for these electrolytes:

- Sodium = 130 – 150 mmol/L (millimoles per liter)
- Chloride = 98- 110 mmol/L
- Potassium = 3.5 – 5.1 mmol/L
- Calcium (ionized, adult) = 1.03 – 1.23 mmol/L
- Inorganic phosphorus = 0.78 – 1.42 mmol/L

These values should be maintained for homeostasis to occur. This is true with the other vital substances that include: glucose, cholesterol, creatinine, triglycerides, urea, and uric acid. There are still various substances in the blood that have to be maintained at their normal levels for your body to achieve homeostasis.

Normal blood pressure

Without other complications, your blood pressure (BP) will remain normal because the substances that can affect its rise and fall are within normal concentrations. "Where sodium is, water follows" is a simple way of explaining this condition. Hence, when your sodium level is normal, your water level tends to be normal also, preventing hypertension. A normal blood pressure will ascertain that your body's systems are safe from destruction; that your organs won't be damaged by your elevated blood pressure.

The US National Heart, Lung and Blood Institute (NHLBI) has established that a normal blood pressure for adults aged 18 and above, is 120/80. 120 is the systolic pressure, and 80 is the diastolic pressure. A blood pressure of 140/90 is categorized as hypertension. NHLBI disclosed that the systolic represents the pressure as the heart beats, whereas, the diastolic indicates the pressure as the heart relaxes between beats. Get your BP daily and record the results to monitor it. It pays to be alert when it comes to your health.

These are the major health benefits of low salt consumption; the unhealthy symptoms will disappear gradually. Less salt intake indicates a healthier body.

Chapter 3: How To Reduce Your Salt Consumption

Reducing your salt consumption may be difficult for you if you're addicted to its savory taste. It's not a gigantic task, however, the minute you are aware of the destructive action of this seemingly harmless substance in your body. Resolve to reduce your salt ingestion, and you're halfway there. The cliché "what the mind can conceive, the body can achieve" is still a good thought to remember. If at first you don't succeed, try and try again until you achieve your goal. Your health is on the line, so be persistent in pursuing your goal.

You can implement the techniques mentioned below to start your quest towards salt reduction in your diet.

Learn how to appreciate foods with less salt

The first step is to make a conscious effort to "re-educate" your palate. Learn how to appreciate less salty foods. At first, this may seem impossible, especially if you're used to salty foods. The knowledge that these foods are damaging to your health will prompt you to avoid them. Inculcate the value of good health so you can move forward with this goal. Your tongue needs getting used to foods without salt, hence, be patient and stand firm with your correct decision. Be resourceful. Experiment with fruits and a variety of vegetable recipes to acquire a healthy "new taste." You might find out to your surprise that cooking unsalted foods brings out their natural flavors. Some vegetable dishes you can cook this way are these:

- Boiled or Broiled cabbage – simply boil the cabbage in water until tender. Eat it, as it is. You can drink, as soup, the water where you boiled the cabbage. You can add string beans and potatoes to the cabbage, as well. Don't add any condiments. Boiling or broiling vegetable is the simplest and quickest way to prepare vegetable dishes.

- Roasted eggplant – Roast eggplants and skin them. Slice onions and tomatoes into thin slices. Eat the eggplants with the onions and tomatoes. You don't need spices or condiments either. Savor slowly to appreciate the complex natural flavors.

Read labels of food products before buying or eating

Each time you buy your food, take time to read the label. The US Food and Drug Administration (FDA) has required proper labeling through the Federal Food, Drug, and Cosmetic Act. Select food products that have low sodium content. Products with 5% sodium concentration are considered low in sodium. You have to take note of the amount of sodium allowable in your diet. Remember that your body needs a little amount of sodium too, because sodium has important functions in your body. Furthermore, you need potassium, because this electrolyte aids in lowering your sodium concentration. If you opt for natural fruits and vegetables, you won't have to read the labels; they also provide a number of health benefits.

Avoid pre-packaged, preserved foods, or canned goods

Pre-packaged, preserved foods and canned goods are rich sources of salt, so avoid them like the plague. They're ticking time bombs ready to explode inside your body to destroy your physiologic balance. Prefer freshly prepared, low salt dishes, because you could control the amount of salt in the dishes. In instances that you can't avoid fast foods, you can request for a no-salt or low-salt dish from the establishment's chef. Most fast food chains accommodate this request. There are always ways to solve problems.

Use alternative flavoring condiments

Instead of using salt, you can use alternative flavoring condiments such as herbs and spices. Herbs and spices lend flavor to your dish without endangering your health. You can use any of the following condiments:

- Celery seeds
- Vanilla
- Pepper
- Garlic powder
- Cilantro
- Rosemary
- Cinnamon
- Marjoram
- Onion powder
- Thyme
- Bay leaf
- Oregano
- Almond
- Basil
- Curry
- Paprika
- Dry mustard

Watch out for non-salty tasting but sodium-rich foods

You have to watch out for those sodium-rich foods which don't actually taste salty. Foods with monosodium glutamate or MSG and baking soda are examples of these. Other non-salty tasting but sodium-rich foods include:

- Canned goods
- Pickled foods
- Cured meat
- Dressings
- Some types of bread
- Frozen meat (hotdogs, ham)
- Frozen meals
- Cheese
- Cereals
- Monosodium glutamate (MSG)

Eat more fruits and vegetables

Eat veggies and fruits; they're essential to your good health. Strive to consume 2-3 servings of fruits or vegetables per day. They are rich in phytochemicals, anti-toxins, vitamins and minerals. Doctors recommend them for most illnesses because they enhance the body's metabolism and excretion of waste products. The alkalinity produced by fruits and vegetables counters the acidity produced by most waste products. This aids in the maintenance of the normal blood pH (alkalinity or acidity) of the body, which ranges from 7.35 to 7.45.

Furthermore, other minerals, namely calcium and potassium are derived from fruits and vegetables. Potassium is important in the transmission of nerve impulses and muscle function. It helps maintain normal blood pressure and prevent hypernatremia too. Good sources of potassium are beans, bananas, prunes, raisins, milk, oranges and spinach.

Cook for yourself

This is one of the most effective methods to ensure that your food has low or no sodium content. When you cook your own food, you can control your salt intake by not adding salt to your recipe. You have the option to choose your own low-sodium-content recipes. You can use alternative seasoning by using herbs and spices. Moreover, cooking your own food assures you that it's clean and safe. It will taste better because you prepared it in consideration of your taste preferences.

These are doable strategies that you can follow to reduce your salt consumption. Learn how to adapt them for a healthier you. A healthy lifestyle is what you need to remain disease-free.

Chapter 4: How To Counteract High Sodium Levels In Your System

You can counteract high sodium levels in your system by learning these natural and proven effective methods, and applying them diligently. Of course, it's advisable for you not to wait until you come to this stage. Prevention is still the vital step in avoiding diseases.

Before you can succeed in counteracting high sodium levels, you should understand the principle that the amount of excess sodium in should be equal to the amount of excess sodium out. The excess sodium you have ingested should all be discarded. The salt requirement of a young, healthy person, without any propensity towards hypertension, kidney or cardiac conditions is below 2,300 mg; more than that amount should be excreted from the body. There are medical interventions used in hospitals to manage hypernatremia, but if your hypernatremia is only due to your salt intake, then there's no need for medical treatment. In cases when hypernatremia is due to an underlying illness, a visit to the doctor is needed.

Here are useful methods in counteracting hypernatremia due to increased salt ingestion:

Hydrate yourself properly

You can counteract hypernatremia by diluting your blood with water. It's like adding tonic water to vodka when preparing a glass of alcoholic drink to lessen the concentration of alcohol. Since it's difficult to remove the salt from your body, you add something to dilute it with, and water is the safest and best diluent for the body. The body requires at least 8 glasses of water daily; hence, you have to drink more to dilute the salt in your blood. While diluting and dissolving the salt in your blood, water will help in salt excretion too, through your kidneys.

Your body cells function well when they are sufficiently hydrated. This facilitates your physiologic functions, including excretion. Water is considered a universal solvent and your body is composed of 60%-70% water. With sufficient water in your cells, these are accomplished:

- Prompt excretion of waste products
- Prevention of the accumulation of salt and other crystals in the kidneys or in the genitourinary tract
- Nourishment of cells and tissues - your cells need to drink just like you need to
- Dissolution and elimination of toxic substances
- Conversion of substances to soluble forms
- Participation in major physiologic and biochemical reactions – water is an active participant in the bicarbonate (HCO_3) and carbonic acid (H_2CO_3) formation. These two substances take part in the blood pH maintenance, just like sodium.

Exercise to sweat off sodium

While increasing your water intake, you should exercise to induce sweating. Your sweat tastes salty because through your sweat, some of the salt or sodium substances are excreted. This will consequently lower your sodium levels. You have to drink more, though, to ensure that ample water is left for your daily water requirement.

When you sweat and you don't have sufficient water in your system, the opposite can happen, because you're dehydrated. Dehydration causes hypernatremia. This is so because there's nothing left to dilute the salt in your blood. It's in the blood where sodium concentrations/levels are measured. Simultaneously, avoid taking in any salt as you hydrate yourself to make sure that the salt content being eliminated is from what's already inside you.

Urinate more often

Increasing your water ingestion will also increase your micturition or urination. There's nothing to worry about. That's fine, as long as you keep hydrating yourself. Drink, drink, and drink. The amount of water you lost through your urine should be replaced promptly through your water intake. The principle is the same as sweating. Urinate to remove salt from your system but drink copious amounts of water to hydrate your cells. It's the same as washing off the salt from your body with water.

The accumulation of salt and crystals in the urinary bladder and the kidneys is greatly reduced when it is washed away promptly with water. The more the salt and crystals accumulate, the easier they can solidify and form stones.

Take in more potassium

Potassium helps stabilize sodium levels in your blood. This essential electrolyte prevents sodium from accumulating by taking the place of sodium. Potassium has an inverse relationship with sodium. Potassium comes from fruits and vegetables mentioned in chapter 3.

Potassium doesn't only aid in decreasing sodium concentration, it also participates in important biochemical reactions because it's the major intracellular electrolyte. It acts as a co-factor for certain enzymatic reactions; it aids in the transmission of nerve impulses; it has a vital role in your heart contraction and H^+ concentration; and is also in charge of the regulation of neuromuscular excitability.

The important fact to remember is that your body doesn't need large amounts of salt; therefore, you should refrain from its habitual use, and get rid of any excess salt in your body.

Chapter 5: The Low Sodium Version Of A Few Traditional American Recipes

Don't worry; you still can eat those tasty dishes. You just have to learn how to prepare their low sodium versions. Lowering your sodium intake doesn't necessarily mean eating bland foods. Learn how to be ingenious and resourceful in cooking and preparing your food. Using unsalted butter and low-sodium cheese are some notable strategies you can use.

To help you with this healthy endeavor, here are three traditional American recipes with low sodium content that you can cook at home.

Potato Salad With Bacon

Ingredients

- 10 slices bacon
- 6 pcs of medium-sized potatoes
- 3 stalks of celery
- Sprinkle of parsley or dill
- 3 pcs Tarragon
- 4 tablespoons vinegar
- ½ teaspoon garlic powder
- ½ cup mayonnaise

Procedure

Step 1 - Wash the ingredients carefully with water.

Step 2 - Cook the bacon and potatoes in separate containers until tender.

Step 3 - After tender, slice the potatoes into ¼ cubes and the bacon into ¼ inch pieces.

Step 4 - Put all the ingredients in one container and mix.

Step 5 - Serve your potato salad with bacon in appropriate containers.

Fried Chicken And Coleslaw

Ingredients

- ½ pc chicken
- ¼ pc cabbage
- 3 pcs onions
- 4 pcs carrots
- 3 pcs shallots
- 8 pcs coriander
- 10 garlic cloves
- 3 cups lemon juice or orange juice
- 1 tablespoon paprika
- 2 tablespoon black pepper
- 1 cup flour
- 2 cups vegetable oil
- 1 cup low salt mayonnaise

Procedure

Step 1 - Marinate the chicken overnight with lemon juice or orange juice, after adding the coriander, garlic and shallots. Refrigerate the preparation.

Step 2 - Prepare the chicken coating by mixing the flour with 1 tablespoon of black pepper and paprika.

Step 3 - Roll the marinated chicken into the prepared coating until evenly coated.

Step 4 - Heat the frying pan or oven and add sufficient vegetable oil to cook your chicken evenly; it should be deep fried. Heat the vegetable oil until sufficiently hot, before adding the chicken.

Step 5 - Deep fry the coated chicken until tender. Make sure you cook both sides. You can use your oven if it is more convenient.

Step 6 - Prepare your coleslaw by washing the cabbage, carrots and onions. Slice them into thin pieces.

Step 7 - Place the sliced cabbage, carrots and onions into a sufficient container and add the mayonnaise and 1 tablespoon of black pepper. Mix thoroughly.

Step 8 - Serve the coleslaw together with the fried chicken.

Barbecue Ribs

Ingredients

- 10 pcs pork spare ribs
- 4 garlic cloves
- 1 medium-sized onion
- 3 tablespoon white vinegar
- 3 tablespoon olive oil
- ½ cup brown sugar
- ½ teaspoon black pepper
- ½ teaspoon cumin
- ½ teaspoon thyme
- 6 pieces tomatoes

Procedure

Step 1 - Prepare the barbecue sauce by chopping the ingredients into thin, small pieces.

Step 2 - Sauté the garlic first, add the onions, and then the tomatoes.

Step 3 - Add the rest of the ingredients and mix. Heat until it boils.

Step 4 - Cover and let the preparation simmer, stirring now and then, to your desired consistency.

Step 5 - Barbecue the spare ribs, taking care not to char them, by brushing them evenly with the barbecue sauce every 3- 5 minutes. Cook until tender.

General Cooking Pointers

- Wash your vegetables and meat thoroughly before slicing them. Numerous pathogenic bacteria come from dirty food.
- Don't overcook the veggies. Cook them just right. They taste the best when not overcooked or raw.
- Use olive oil in place of meat oil because it's healthier.
- Boil carrots in cinnamon to make them tastier.
- Pineapple juice can be used in place of lemon or orange juice.
- Use spices and herbs in place of salt, when a recipe requires salt.
- For the barbecue ribs, avoid charring the meat because the National Cancer Institute has disclosed that the component of charred meat, namely heterocyclic amines (HCAs) and polycyclic aromatic hydrocarbons (PAHs) caused cancer in laboratory rats.
- Protect your food from outside contamination with microorganisms and toxins by covering your food at all times.

The amount of each ingredient will vary according to your taste. You can vary the amount of the ingredients. You can also add more ingredients such as sage and thyme. If you want to add salt, use the alternatives given in chapter 3, or add sparingly.

Even without adding table salt to your dishes, you can ingest salt from the ingredients of your meals. Double check these ingredients before using them. Choose fresh preparations instead of processed products. Cook your favorite dish, taking conscious effort not to add salt needlessly. Succulent dishes can still be prepared without salt.

Chapter 6: Low Sodium Breakfast Recipes

Breads And Muffins

Breads are a wonderful part of the breakfast platter and there's plenty of variety offered by simply adding new ingredients to the core recipe. When breads are made in smaller molds then they are known as muffins, which are also very popular for their easy preparation and smaller size. Here are some of the choicest breads and muffins, each with an appealing twist to it.

Apple Cinnamon Bread

A traditional favorite is the Apple Cinnamon Bread, which can be easily prepared in large quantities and be frozen in a tightly sealed plastic bag. The bread can also be stored at room temperature for up to four days in a plastic bag. This recipe can be used to make single slice servings for 8 persons and the ingredients can be doubled if larger quantity is desired but then two separate loaf pans must be used for the baking process.

Preparation Time: 30 minutes

Cooking Time: 60 minutes

Servings: Single slice serving for 8 people
Sodium Value per serving: 308mg

Ingredients

- ☐ White wheat flour ¾ cup
- ☐ All-purpose white flour 1 ¼ cups
- ☐ Baking powder 2 tsp
- ☐ Baking soda ½ tsp
- ☐ Pure vanilla essence ½ tsp
- ☐ Sweet stevia or Splenda 2/3 cup
- ☐ Salt ¼ tsp
- ☐ Ground cinnamon 1 tsp + ¼ tsp separate
- ☐ Pecans ¼ cup (coarsely chopped)
- ☐ Maple syrup 2 tsp
- ☐ Wheat germ ¼ cup
- ☐ Egg yolk 1 large sized
- ☐ Egg whites 3 large sized
- ☐ Canola oil 1 tsp
- ☐ Apples 2 cups (peeled, cored and grated)
- ☐ Apple sauce (unsweetened) ½ cup
- ☐ Buttermilk (low fat) ½ cup

Directions

Preheat oven to 350☐F and take a 1½ quart loaf pan having an oblong shape. It would be best to line it with non-stick foil. The pan can be either glass Pyrex or a thick metal pan.

First combine the maple syrup with the pecans and ¼ tsp cinnamon, stirring until the mixture is blended completely and then set it aside. The next step is to whisk the egg yolk with either a hand whisk or electric beater till it becomes smooth. Add the canola oil and keep whisking until it is smooth. Then slowly add in batches the Z-sweet or Splenda, applesauce and vanilla essence to the yolk mixture until it falls off the whisk in ribbons. Beat the egg whites in a separate bowl till they become frothy and white. Try to avoid over-beating as stiff peaks are not required.

Take all the dry ingredients i.e. the wheat germ, all-purpose flour, whole wheat flour, baking soda, baking powder, salt and cinnamon powder and sift them into a large mixing bowl. Next, fold in the egg yolk mixture into the dry mixture and it would be preferable to do it with a spoon or fork to ensure proper blending. Once it is done, then the grated apples can be added. After that the buttermilk is to be folded in until the mixture is smooth. Lastly the frothed egg whites are to be folded into the mixture.

After all the mixing is done, the batter is then to be poured into the lined loaf pan and topped evenly with the pecan and maple syrup mixture. Then place the dish in the pre-heated oven and bake for an hour. Once done, remove from the oven and then allow it to cool in the dish for 10 minutes before removing from dish.

Gingerbread

The zingy taste of ginger in bread makes it a delightful treat for both adults and kids. This bread can be shaped in interesting ways to suit the occasion. It lasts for three to four days and can be sealed in a tight plastic bag for being frozen. It needs to be re-heated mildly to keep the ginger taste pleasant. This recipe can be doubled but then two separate loaf pans will be required for baking.

Preparation Time: 20 minutes

Cooking Time: 50 minutes

Servings: Single slice serving for 8 people

Sodium Value per serving: 347mg

Ingredients

☐ Egg Yolk 1 large sized

☐ Canola Oil 1 tsp

☐ Sweet Stevia or Splenda ½ cup

☐ Canned Pumpkin ½ cup

☐ Unsweetened Applesauce ½ cup

☐ Pure Vanilla Extract ½ tsp

☐ Molasses 2 Tbsp

☐ Egg Whites 3 large sized

☐ All Purpose Flour 1 ¼ cup

☐ Whole Wheat Flour ¾ cup

☐ Salt ¼ tsp

☐ Baking Powder 2 tsp

☐ Baking Soda ½ tsp

☐ Ground Cinnamon 1 tsp

☐ Ground Ginger 2 tsp

☐ Wheat Germ ¼ cup

☐ LowFat Buttermilk ½ cup

Directions

Preheat the oven to 350°F and take an oblong shaped loaf pan (preferably a Pyrex glass one). Use nonstick baking foil to line the pan.

First whisk the egg yolk until takes the form of a smooth paste, then add the canola oil and whisk some more. Then in the next step come the Splenda or Z-sweet, unsweetened apple sauce, vanilla extract and canned pumpkin to make a thick and smooth mixture. Lastly, you need to slowly whisk the molasses into the mixture.

Take an electric beater and beat the beat the egg whites until then turn into a white frothy mixture but try to avoid over-beating and making stiff peaks of the whites.

Take the flours, salt, cinnamon, ground ginger, wheat germ, baking soda and baking powder ad sift them into a large mixing bowl. Then with a spoon or fork fold in the creamed yolk mixture. Slowly add buttermilk into the mixture and keep folding gently till it becomes smooth.

As a final step, add the frothy egg whites into the batter and fold it some more till it becomes smooth.

Take the lined loaf pan and pour the mixture into it. Then bake it in the pre-heated oven for approximately 50 minutes. Decorate it after it has cooled completely.

Date Nut Quickbread

Dates are a very good source of energy and provide a person with instant vitality. Putting dates in bread give it a lovely sweet taste but also make a good energy food. This recipe can be doubled easily. The bread can be stored in a plastic wrapper for up to 4 days and can be frozen quite well too.

Preparation Time: 20 minutes

Cooking Time: 50 minutes

Servings: Single slice serving for 8 people

Sodium Value per serving: 304mg

Ingredients

☐ Chopped Dates ½ cup

☐ Boiling Water ½ cup

☐ Egg Yolk 1 large

☐ Canola Oil 1 tsp

☐ Sweet Stevia or Splenda ½ cup

☐ Unsweetened Applesauce ½ cup

☐ Pure Vanilla Extract ½ cup

☐ Molasses 1 Tbsp

☐ Egg Whites 3 large

☐ All Purpose Flour 1 ¼ cup

☐ Whole Wheat Flour ¾ cup

☐ Salt ¼ tsp

☐ Baking Powder 2 tsp

☐ Baking Soda ½ tsp
☐ Ground Cinnamon 1 tsp
☐ Chopped Pecans ½ cup
☐ Wheat Germ ¼ cup
☐ LowFat Buttermilk ¼ cup

Directions

Preheat the oven to 350°F and take an oblong shaped loaf pan (preferably a Pyrex glass one). Use nonstick baking foil to line the pan.

First of all you have to put the dates in a bowl and pour boiling water over them. Leave the dates in the water for at least 15 minutes so that they soften. Stir them once or twice. Then remove them from the water and pat them dry with a paper towel.

Then you have to whisk the egg yolk until takes the form of a smooth paste, then add the canola oil and whisk some more. Then in the next step come the Splenda or Z-sweet, unsweetened apple sauce, vanilla extract and softened dates to make a thick and smooth mixture. Lastly, you need to slowly whisk the molasses into the mixture.

Take an electric beater and beat the beat the egg whites until then turn into a white frothy mixture but try to avoid over-beating and making stiff peaks of the whites.

Take the flours, salt, cinnamon, wheat germ, baking soda and baking powder ad sift them into a large mixing bowl. Then with a spoon or fork fold in the creamed yolk mixture. Add the pecans and stir well to mix them up.

Slowly add buttermilk into the mixture and keep folding gently till it becomes smooth. As a final step, add the frothy egg whites into the batter and fold it some more till it becomes smooth.

Take the lined loaf pan and pour the mixture into it. Then bake it in the pre-heated oven for approximately 50 minutes. Decorate it after it has cooled completely.

Banana Nut Bread

This healthy bread is a kids' favorite due to the banana flavor and can be used as a kiddy treat. It is a good addition in an adult's breakfast menu as well. The recipe has common ingredients with the Apple Cinnamon Bread and just needs a few alterations in the preparation process. It can also be stored at room temperature up to 4 days in a plastic bag and can be frozen in a tightly sealed plastic bag. It needs to be re-heated gently though. This recipe can be doubled but two separate loaf pans must be used for baking then.

Preparation Time: 35 minutes

Cooking Time: 55 minutes

Servings: Single slice serving for 8 people
Sodium per Serving: 301mg

Ingredients

☐ Whole wheat flour ¾ cup

☐ All purpose white flour 1 ¼ cups

☐ Baking powder 2 tsp

☐ Baking soda ½ tsp

☐ Pure vanilla essence ½ tsp

☐ Sweet stevia or Splenda 2/3 cup

☐ Salt   ¼ tsp

☐ Ground cinnamon ½ tsp

☐ Pecans ½ cup (coarsely chopped)

☐ Wheat germ ¼ cup

- ☐ Egg yolk 1 large
- ☐ Egg whites 3 large
- ☐ Canola oil ½ tsp
- ☐ Bananas 2 medium sized and very ripe (mashed)
- ☐ Ground nutmeg ¼ tsp
- ☐ Buttermilk (low fat) ¼ cup
- ☐ Light Brown Sugar 2 tsp

Directions

Preheat oven to 350☐F and take a 1 ½ quart loaf pan having an oblong shape. It would be best to line it with non-stick foil. The pan can be either glass Pyrex or a thick metal pan.

The first step is to whisk the egg yolk with either a hand whisk or electric beater till it becomes smooth. Add the canola oil and keep whisking until it is smooth. Then slowly add the mashed bananas and mix it up till it becomes a smooth paste. The next step is to add the Z-sweet or Splenda and vanilla essence to the yolk mixture until it falls off the whisk in ribbons. Beat the egg whites in a separate bowl till they become frothy and white. Try to avoid over-beating as stiff peaks are not required.

Take all the dry ingredients i.e. the wheat germ, all-purpose flour, whole wheat flour, baking soda, baking powder, salt, nutmeg and cinnamon powder and sift them into a large mixing bowl. Next, gently fold in the egg yolk mixture into the dry mixture and it would be preferable to do it with a spoon or fork to ensure proper blending. Then add the chopped pecans to the mixture. Once it is done, the frothed egg whites are to be folded into the mixture to get a smooth consistency.In the end, the buttermilk is to be folded in until it completely blends in.

After all the mixing is done, the batter is then to be poured into the lined loaf pan and sprinkled evenly with the light brown sugar. Then place the dish in the pre-heated oven and bake for around 55 minutes. Once done, remove from the oven and then allow it to cool in the dish for 10 minutes before removing from dish.

Banana Nut Muffin

The banana nut muffin is the junior version of the bread and it requires a little less time and effort. This healthy muffin can last for nearly two days in a plastic bag at room temperature and freezes even better than the bread, if frozen in a tightly sealed plastic bag.

Preparation Time: 15 minutes

Cooking Time: 20 minutes

Servings: Single muffin serving for 6 people

Sodium per Serving: 251mg

Ingredients

☐ Whole wheat flor ½ cup

☐ All purpose white flour 1 cup

☐ Baking powder 1tsp

☐ Baking soda ¼ tsp

☐ Pure vanilla essence½ tsp

☐ Sweet stevia or Splenda ½ cup

☐ Salt ¼ tsp

☐ Ground cinnamon½ tsp

☐ Pecans ¼ cup (coarsely chopped)

☐ Wheat germ 2 tbsp

☐ Egg 1 large (separated)

☐ Canola oil 2tsp

☐ Bananas 1 large sized and very ripe (mashed)

☐ Ground nutmeg ¼tsp

☐Buttermilk (low fat)¼ cup

☐Light Brown Sugar2 tsp

Directions

Preheat the oven to 375☐F. The separated egg yolk and canola oil are to be whisked together until a creamy mixture forms. A handheld whisk would be preferable. The mashed bananas are the next ingredient to go into the mixture. Next to go in, are the vanilla essence and Splenda/stevia. After they have been blended, the pecans are to be folded in.

The two flours, wheat germ, nutmeg, cinnamon, baking powder, baking soda and salt must be sifted together into a large mixing bowl. Then the creamed batter is to be folded into the dry mixture, to get dry dough. With the help of an electric beater, beat the egg white till it becomes foamy and almost triple in volume. Then fold that into the batter as well. The last ingredient is the buttermilk, which will give the dough the proper texture. The buttermilk has to be folded in until the dough is just blended (no need for over blending).

A standard sized muffin tin with 6 cups is needed. It can either be greased or lined with paper liners. Most bakery shops have beautiful colored paper liners, which are attractive for kids. Spoon the mixture evenly into each cup and leave some space for the leavening of the muffin. Place the muffin tin in the preheated oven and bake for nearly 20 minutes. You can check if the muffins cook early by inserting a toothpick into the muffin and see if it comes out clean. Turn out the muffins on a wire rack and cool them completely before serving.

Blueberry Muffin

The delightful taste of blueberries makes this muffin simply amazing and has the additional zing of yogurt to it as well. This recipe can be multiplied according to requirement and is relatively easy to make. These muffins can also be frozen in a tightly sealed plastic bag and will keep for nearly two days when stored in a plastic bag.

Preparation Time: 15 minutes

Cooking Time: 15 minutes

Serving: Single muffin serving for 6 people

Sodium per Serving: 265 mg

Ingredients

☐ All purpose white flour 1 cup

☐ Whole wheat flour½ cup

☐ Wheat germ 2 tbsp

☐ Canola oil 2 tsp

☐ Sweet stevia or Splenda ½ cup

☐ Egg 1 large sized (separated)

☐ No-fat yogurt 2 tbsp

☐ Pure vanilla extract½ tsp

☐ Salt ¼ tsp

☐ Baking powder 1 tsp

☐ Baking soda ¼tsp

☐ Lowfat buttermilk ½ cup

☐ Blueberries ½cup

Directions

Preheat oven to 375☐F. First beat the egg yolk and canola oil together to make the creamy mixture and then add the stevia or Splenda, vanilla extract and yogurt to it – whisking until the mixture is smooth and holds together. Then whisk the egg white until it is foamy and white.

Sift together the flours, wheat germ, salt, baking soda and baking powder. Then in a large mixing bowl fold the creamed egg yolk mix with the dry mixture. Add the buttermilk in batches to the batter, folding it gently until it is smooth and well blended.

Then fold in the foamy egg whites and then lastly the blueberries. The batter must not be over-mixed and you must stop as soon as it is smooth. A 6 cup muffin tin is to be lined with paper liners and then the batter is poured in equal mounts into each cup. Place the tin in the preheated oven and bake for 12 to 15 minutes. Make sure the muffins are cooled on a wire rack before serving.

Bran Muffin

It is important to have plenty of fiber in your daily diet and what better option than adding a bran muffin to your early morning meal. This recipe is ideal for people who are watching their weight and are in favor of a healthy breakfast due to the low amount of fat. These muffins will keep only for one day and can be frozen after being wrapped individually in plastic wrap. Their re-heating is a bit tricky because it requires them to be thawed out for nearly 20 minutes and then reheated in a moderately hot oven.

Preparation Time: 10 minutes

Cooking Time: 20 minutes

Serving: Single muffin serving for 8 people
Sodium per Serving: 329 mg

Ingredients

☐ All purpose white flour 1 cup

☐ Kellog's All Bran Flakes 1 ½ cups

☐ Splenda or Z-sweet stevia ½ cup

☐ Baking powder 2 ½ tsp

☐ 2% milk 1 cup

☐ Salt ½ cup

☐ Egg 1 large sized

☐ Grape seed oil 1 tbsp

☐ Unsweetened applesauce ¼ cup

Directions

Preheat the oven to 375□F. Take the bran and mix it with the milk in a bowl. Leave the bran to soften in the milk for 20 minutes. While the bran is softening, you can sift together the flour, Splenda/stevia, salt and baking powder into a large mixing bowl. Then add the softened bran mixture to the dry mixture and whisk them. Finally add the last three ingredients into the batter and whisk until it has a smooth consistency. Once again, it is advisable not to over mix because then the muffins do not rise properly while baking.

In this case a 12 cup muffin tray is required but only 8 of the cups need to be lined with paper liners of your choice. The batter needs to fill 2/3 of each cup in order to get a nice puffy crown for the muffins. Bake in the pre-heated oven for around 20 minutes and do check if a toothpick comes out clean after 15 minutes. You do not want to burn your muffins.

Carrot Muffin

Adding vegetables to muffins is a great way to smuggle veggies into kids' diet! The muffins taste good and are a very healthy way of starting the day. This recipe can be multiplied twice and the muffins can be prepared in large numbers and stored for future use by being frozen in tightly sealed plastic wrappers. They have to be reheated gently to ensure the carrots don't lose their color. The muffins can be stored at room temperature for nearly 2 days.

Preparation Time: 15 minutes

Cooking Time: 15 minutes

Serving: Single muffin serving for 6 people

Sodium per Serving: 278 mg

Ingredients

☐ Egg 1 large sized (separated)

☐ Canola Oil 2 tsp

☐ Sweet Stevia or Splenda ½ cup

☐ Nor-Fat Yogurt 2 Tbsp

☐ Pure Vanilla Essence ½ tsp

☐ All Purpose White Flour 1 cup

☐ Whole Wheat Flour ½ cup

☐ Salt ¼ tsp

☐ Baking Powder 1 tsp

☐ Baking Soda ¼ tsp

☐ Ground Cinnamon ½ tsp

☐ Ground Nutmeg ¼tsp

☐ Carrots (Peeled and Shredded)1 cup

☐ Oatmeal (Quick, Not Instant)¼ cup

☐ LowFat Buttermilk ½ cup

Directions

Preheat the oven to 375☐F. Take the separated egg white and whisk it into a frothy foamy mixture. Then add the canola oil into it slowly as you whisk. Next to go in, are the vanilla essence, egg yolk, yogurt and Splenda/stevia. Keep on whisking till the mixture is smooth.

The two flours, nutmeg, cinnamon, baking powder, baking soda and salt must be sifted together into a large mixing bowl. You should sprinkle the oatmeal flakes over the dry mixture. Then the creamed batter is to be folded into the dry mixture, to get dry dough.

Then add the carrots while slowly folding the mixture. The last ingredient is the buttermilk and it has to be folded in until the dough is just blended (no need for over blending).

A standard sized muffin tin with 6 cups is needed. It can either be greased or lined with paper liners. Spoon the mixture evenly into each cup and place it in the preheated oven and bake from 12-15 minutes. Turn out the muffins on a wire rack and cool them completely before serving.

Cornbread Muffin

The pure fiber in a cornbread muffin is a good start for the digestive system. This recipe is simple and quite quick to prepare and cook. It is advisable to consume these muffins within one day and if frozen then you have to wrap each muffin individually in plastic wrap. To re-heat, first thaw the muffins for 20 minutes, then slice each muffin in half and place in an oven that has been preheated at 300°F. Try not to multiply the recipe but rather make the muffins in separate batches for good results.

Preparation Time: 10 minutes

Cooking Time: 15 minutes

Serving: Single muffin serving for 12 people

Sodium per Serving: 225 mg

Ingredients

☐ Yellow Cornmeal ¾ cup

☐ All Purpose Flour 1 cup

☐ Sugar 1/3 cup

☐ Baking Powder 1 Tbsp

☐ Salt ½ tsp

☐ Nor-Fat Buttermilk 1 cup

☐ Egg 1 large sized (separated)

☐ Unsalted Butter 1 Tbsp

Directions

Preheat the oven to 325°F and line a large 12-pocket muffin tin with paper liners.

Thoroughly mix all the ingredients in a large mixing bowl and allow the mixture to stand for around ten minutes.

Pour the mixture evenly into the muffin cups and bake in the oven for nearly 15 minutes. The muffins should be having a golden crown when ready. Turn out the muffins on a wire rack and cool before serving.

Orange Almond Muffins

This recipe adds the zesty flavor of oranges to the regular muffin and gives you a refreshing experience. The muffins will keep for around four days and can be frozen if stored in a tightly sealed plastic bag. You can double this recipe if you wish.

Preparation Time: 15 minutes

Cooking Time: 22 minutes

Serving: Single muffin serving for 6 people

Sodium per Serving: 258 mg

Ingredients

☐ Egg Separated 1 large

☐ Canola Oil 1 tsp

☐ Sweet Stevia or Splenda ½ cup

☐ NorFat Yogurt 2 Tbsp

☐ Pure Almond Extract 1 ½ tsp

☐ All Purpose Flour 1 cup

☐ Whole Wheat Flour ½ cup

☐ Salt ¼ tsp

☐ Baking Powder 1 tsp

☐ Baking Soda 1 tsp

☐ Wheat Germ 2 Tbsp

☐ Orange Zest 1 tsp

☐ Slvered Blanched Almonds ½ cup

☐ LowFat Buttermilk ¼ cup

☐ Orange Juice 1/3 cup

☐ Light Brown Sugar 2 tsp

Directions

Preheat oven to 375☐F. First beat the egg yolk and canola oil together to make the creamy mixture and then add the stevia or Splenda, almond extract and yogurt to it – whisking until the mixture is smooth and holds together. Then whisk the egg white until it is foamy and white.

Sift together the flours, wheat germ, salt, baking soda and baking powder. Then place the dry ingredients in a large mixing bowl and add the orange zest and ¼ cup of almonds (reserving the rest for decoration). Then fold the creamed egg yolk mix with the dry mixture. Then fold in the foamy egg whites to get a smooth batter. Add the buttermilk and orange juice in batches to the batter, folding it gently until it is smooth and well blended.

The batter must not be over-mixed and you must stop as soon as it is smooth. A 6 cup muffin tin is to be lined with paper liners and then the batter is poured in equal mounts into each cup. Sprinkle the brown sugar and remaining almonds on top of the cups. Place the tin in the preheated oven and bake for 20 to 22 minutes. Make sure the muffins are cooled on a wire rack before serving.

Orange Blueberry Scones

Scones can be served at breakfast and at tea-time. These scones can be prepared in large numbers and kept for nearly three days at room temperature in a plastic bag. They can also be kept in the refrigerator for quite a few days. This recipe can be doubled without any problems.

Preparation Time: 20 minutes

Cooking Time: 18 minutes

Serving: Single one serving for 8 people

Sodium per Serving: 297 mg

Ingredients

☐ All Purpose Flour 2 cups

☐ Light Brown Sugar ¼ cup

☐ Baking Powder 2 tsp

☐ Salt ½ tsp

☐ Unsalted Butter (Softened) 2 Tbsp

☐ Fresh grated Orange peel 1 tsp

☐ Orange Juice ¼ cup

☐ NorFat Buttermilk ¾ cup

☐ Blueberries ¼ cup

☐ NorFat Buttermilk 2 Tbsp

☐ Light Brown Sugar 1 Tbsp

Directions

Preheat the oven to a high temperature of 425°F. First of all sift together the flour, salt, baking powder and sugar in a large mixing bowl. Then use your hands to rub in the chopped and softened butter. You can also use a fork or pastry knife to do the same thing. The end result should be a mixture that looks like bread crumbs. Now this is ready for addition of the orange juice and orange peel.

Knead the dough with your hands or with the help of a rubber spatula, while the addition of the orange juice and orange peel. Then continue the kneading and add the buttermilk. Now this will become a sticky kind of dough.

With care add the blueberries into this dough and try not to knead too much or the berries with pop. Take small portions of the dough and shape them into little triangles. You should end up with eight triangles. Grease a non-stick baking tray and lay out all the scones on it.

The last step is to brush the top of each scone with a mixture of the remaining 2 tbsp buttermilk and 1 tbsp brown sugar. You can use a pastry brush to do the job. Bake for fifteen to twenty minutes in the preheated oven. The scones are golden colored when they are done.

Orange Cranberry Muffins

The sweetness of cranberries when combined with the zing of oranges in a muffin can be a real treat to eat. This recipe can be doubled and tripled. The muffins will stay fresh for nearly 3 days when stored in a plastic bag. When sealed tightly, they can be frozen quite well.

Preparation Time: 15 minutes

Cooking Time: 15 minutes

Serving: Single muffin serving for 6 people

Sodium per Serving: 257 mg

Ingredients

☐ Egg (Separated) 1 large

☐ Canola Oil 2 tsp

☐ Sweet Stevia or Splenda ½ cup

☐ No-Fat Yogurt 2 Tbsp

☐ Reduced-Fat Sour Cream 2 Tbsp

☐ Pure Vanilla Extract ½ tsp

☐ All Purpose White Flour 1 cup

☐ Whole Wheat Flour ½ cup

☐ Salt ¼ tsp

☐ Baking Powder 1 tsp

☐ Baking Soda ¼ tsp

☐ Cranberries 1/3 cup

☐ Wheat Germ 2 Tbsp

☐ Low-Fat Buttermilk ¼ cup

☐ Orange Jice ¼ cup

☐ Orange Zest 1 tsp

Directions

Preheat the oven to 375☐F. Take the separated egg white and whisk it into a frothy foamy mixture. Then add the canola oil into it slowly as you whisk. Next to go in, are the vanilla essence, sour cream, egg yolk, yogurt and Splenda/stevia. Keep on whisking till the mixture is smooth.

The two flours, baking powder, baking soda and salt must be sifted together into a large mixing bowl. You should carefully mix the cranberries into the mixture, so that they do not stick together. Add the wheat germ into the mixture. Then the creamed batter is to be folded into the dry mixture, to get the dough.

The last step is to combine the buttermilk, orange juice and zest and folded in until the dough is just blended (no need for over blending).

A standard sized muffin tin with 6 cups is needed. It can either be greased or lined with paper liners. Spoon the mixture evenly into each cup and place it in the preheated oven and bake from 12-15 minutes. Turn out the muffins on a wire rack and cool them completely before serving.

Lemon Poppy Seed Muffin

The hearty taste of lemon is enough to awaken the senses early in the morning and this muffin is a mouthful when done properly. This recipe can be multiplied twice or thrice. The muffins are good for at least a day in a plastic bag and can be frozen when sealed tightly.

Preparation Time: 15 minutes

Cooking Time: 20 minutes

Serving: Single muffin serving for 6 people

Sodium per Serving: 273 mg

Ingredients

☐ Egg 1 large sized (separated)

☐ Canola Oil 1 tsp

☐ Sweet Stevia or Splenda ½ cup

☐ No-Fat Yogurt 2 Tbsp

☐ Pure Vanilla Extract ½ tsp

☐ Poppy Seeds 2 Tbsp

☐ Lemon Zest 1 Tbsp

☐ Fresh Lemon Juice ¼ cup

☐ All Purpose White Flour 1 cup

☐ Whole Wheat Flour ½ cup

☐ Wheat Germ 2 Tbsp

☐ Salt ¼ tsp

☐ Baking Powder 1 tsp

☐ Baking Soda ¼ tsp

☐ LowFat Buttermilk 1/3 cup

Directions

Preheat the oven to 375☐F. The separated egg yolk and canola oil are to be whisked together until a creamy mixture forms. A handheld whisk would be preferable. Next to go in, are the vanilla essence, poppy seeds, yogurt, lemon zest, lemon juice and Splenda/stevia. Keep on whisking until all the ingredients have blended in completely and the mixture is smooth.

The two flours, baking powder, baking soda and salt must be sifted together into a large mixing bowl. Then the creamed batter is to be folded into the dry mixture, to get dry dough.

Then comes the buttermilk, which will give the dough the proper texture. The buttermilk has to be folded in until the batter is just blended.

With the help of an electric beater, beat the egg white till it becomes foamy and almost triple in volume. Then fold that into the batter as well.

A standard sized muffin tin with 6 cups is needed. It can either be greased or lined with paper liners. Spoon the mixture evenly into each cup and leave some space for the leavening of the muffin. Place the muffin tin in the preheated oven and bake for nearly 20 minutes. Check after 18 minutes if the muffins are done. Turn out the muffins on a wire rack and cool them completely before serving.

Pancakes

The yummy goodness of a pancake can't be beaten with anything else in the breakfast platter. The art of making pancakes is subtle and yet simple. Adding sauces and fruits to the basic pancake recipe can be very gratifying for the taste buds and the stomach!

Pan Baked Apple Pancake

An apple is a favorite fruit for all of us due to its nutritional value and crisp taste, and that is what makes the pan baked apple pancake so merry! This pancake can be stored in the refrigerator once it has been cooled. But you have to wrap it very tightly in plastic wrap.

Preparation Time: 20minutes

Cooking Time: 18 minutes

Serving: ¼ pancake serving for 4 people

Sodium per Serving: 237 mg

Ingredients

☐ Granny Smith 4 MediumApples 2lbs

☐ Unsalted Butter 2 tsp

☐ Splenda or Stevia ½cup

☐ Water ¼ cup

☐ Egg Whites 3 large

☐ Egg Yolk 1 large

☐ NorFat Buttermilk ¾ cup

☐ All Purpose White Flour ¾ cup

☐ Salt ¼ tsp

☐ Splenda or Stevia 2 Tbsp

Directions

Preheat the oven to 425°F. Thinly slice the peeled and core apples. Keep the thickness to approximately 1/8 inch. Then in a large non-stick frying pan or iron skillet, heat the butter and add the Splenda/stevia and water to it till it boils. Add the apples into the pan and keep turning them to cook through. Keep up this process for 15 minutes ad at the end the apples should be of a caramel brown color with very little liquid left.

During the cooking of the apples, take the remainder of the ingredients, except the last 2tsp of butter, and blend them together till a smooth paste forms. Finally pour this mixture over the caramelized apples in the pan. The mixture should cover the apples completely.

Place the pan in the preheated oven and bake for around 18 minutes. The pancake puffs up a bit during cooking and it is done when the top turns light brown. Keep checking after 15 minutes to prevent over-cooking.

Buckwheat Pancake

The cereal-like grain of the buckwheat adds a welcome texture to these pancakes. This recipe can be multiplied as many times as you wish to. But it is best to consume all the pancakes at that time because leftovers can't be stored.

Preparation Time: 10minutes

Cooking Time: 15 minutes

Serving: Double pancake serving for 2 people

Sodium per Serving: 484 mg

Ingredients

☐ Egg Yolk 1 large

☐ Champagne (beer will do) ¼ cup

☐ Milk 2 Tbsp

☐ Buckwheat Flour1/3 cup

☐ Selfrising Flour 1/3 cup

☐ Salt 1/8 tsp

☐ Egg Whites 2 large

☐ Butter 3 tsp

☐ Maple Syrup 2 Tbsp

Directions

Take the champagne and mix the egg yolk and milk into it. Keep on whisking till the mixture is well blended and keep on whisking while you add the buckwheat flour, flour and salt in it.

Using an electric beater beat the egg whites into stiff peaks. Then fold these stiff whites into the batter slowly.

Take a griddle pan and heat it to the extent that water will evaporate immediately if sprayed on it. Melt one teaspoon of butter and quickly drop 1/3 cup of the batter into the pan and rotate the pan to spread it evenly. Flip the pancake over when bubbles appear on the surface and cook for a short while before removing from pan. Repeat the process to get four pancakes. Serve the pancakes while hot and top off with maple syrup and additional butter.

Buttermilk Pancakes

The simple plain pancakes can be served at breakfast or tea time, with difference of condiments. These buttermilk pancakes can be multiplied as many times as desired and it is best to completely consume them within one day because storing them is not possible.

Preparation Time: 5minutes

Cooking Time: 15 minutes

Serving: Double pancake serving for 2 people

Sodium per Serving: 406 mg

Ingredients

☐ All purpose White Flour 2/3 cup

☐ Splenda or Stevia 1 Tbsp

☐ Baking Powder 1 tsp

☐ Norfat Buttermilk 2/3 cup

☐ Egg 1 large

☐ Pure Vanilla extract 1 tsp

☐ Unsalted Butter (Per Serving)1 Tbsp

☐ Pure Maple Syrup (Per Serving) 1 Tbsp

Directions

Sift together the Splenda/stevia, baking powder and flour into a mixing bowl. Combine the buttermilk, vanilla extract and egg in a small jug and slowly whisk this mixture into the dry mixture. Keep on whisking till the mixture forms a thick smooth paste.

Take a non-stick griddle pan and heat t till it is very hot. Then lower the heat and grease it ever so slightly with a pastry brush. Then put a ¼ cup dollop of the batter in the middle of the pan and rotate it to spread out the mixture evenly. Cook one side of the pancake till its surface turns bubbly, then turn it with the help of a spatula. Let the other side cook for around one minute till it is golden brown.

You can serve the pancakes with yogurt and honey or butter it on both sides and serve it with maple syrup.

Frittatas And Egg Related Dishes

Eggs are a time-old traditional part of breakfast menus all around the world. Maybe it is because eggs provide most of the daily requirement of vitamins and have good fats and proteins. This means having an egg in one's diet is a good way to cover maximum nutritional needs. Eggs are cooked in a variety of forms and served in many different ways.

Omelet | Low Sodium Version

Omelets are thinner than frittatas, hence there is no need to bake them and veggies and cheese can be added to experiment with the flavors. This recipe can be multiplied as many times as you desire but then you need to cook in batches.

Preparation Time: 10minutes

Cooking Time: 5 minutes

Serving: Half omelet serving for 2 people

Sodium per Serving: 232 mg

Take a medium sized non stick frying pan and place it over normal heat. Melt the butter in the pan and cook the peppers in it till they are slightly brown but still firm. Remove and set them aside.

Next, take the whites and yolks and whisk them in a mixing bowl. Add water and then season with freshly ground black pepper.

Heat up the pan once again on medium heat and sprinkle it with the basil. Now pour the egg mixture on top of it. Lower the heat a bit and cook slowly. With the help of a spatula, gently fold over the cooked part, so that the rest of the mixture can cook as well. When the eggs are nearly done, align the peppers in a straight line in the center of the omelet and fold it in half to completely cover the peppers. Keep on cooking for two more minutes, and then remove from the pan.

As a finishing touch, sprinkle the cheese over the folded omelet and cut it into two neat portions for serving.

Eggs Benedict

This recipe is best served with Hollandaise sauce and English muffins. The sauce has to be prepared separately, while English muffins are easily available from bakeries. Try to eat the entire prepared dish because it spoils easily. It can be multiplied as many times as you need.

Preparation Time: 5minutes

Cooking Time: 25 minutes

Serving: 1 person

Sodium per Serving: 250 mg

Ingredients

☐ Water 2 quarts

☐ White Wine Vinegar 1 Tbsp

☐ Asparagus Spears 5

☐ English Muffin ½ piece

☐ Egg 1 large

☐ Hollandaise Sauce 2 Tbsp

Directions

Separate the water into two quarts and pour one quart into a medium sized skillet over a moderate flame. Do not bring the water to a full boil but place the asparagus into the water as soon as it seems slightly bubbly. Cook the asparagus spears for nearly five to seven minutes so that they are bright green in color and are just a little floppy. Carefully take the asparagus out of the water but do not drain the water from the pan. Keep the water at poaching stage.

Take the other quart of water in another large skillet and heat it up too. Add vinegar to it and do not let the water reach boiling point. Now place the asparagus back into the first pan.

Here comes the tricky part of poaching the egg. Break the egg into either a teacup or a custard cup. Gently pour the egg into the second pan which has the water and vinegar mixture. The egg should poach nice and slow. While this is taking place, pop one half of the English muffin into the toaster and begin toasting it.

Meanwhile, heat the Hollandaise sauce over a gentle heat and keep stirring it. Do not boil it but keep it hot. If it is too hot then it will spoil the poached egg.

By the time the muffin is toasted properly, the asparagus and egg should also be done. So in order to serve it, you have to place the English muffin smooth side down on a warm serving plate. Then arrange the blanched asparagus over it and trim the spears if you do not like them poking out. Next gently place the poached egg over it and decorate it with the Hollandaise sauce.

Hollandaise Sauce

This sauce can be used as a condiment for the Eggs Benedict but is sure to use it on the same day while it is fresh.

Preparation Time: 5 minutes

Cooking Time: 15 minutes

Serving: 2 tablespoons sized serving for 8 people
Sodium per Serving: 86 mg

Ingredients

☐ Corn Starch 1 ½ Tbsp

☐ 2% Milk 2/3 cup

☐ Unsalted Butter 1 tsp

☐ Fresh Lemon Juice 2 ½ Tbsp

☐ Egg Yolk 1

☐ Salt ¼ tsp

Directions

Mix the cornstarch and cold milk in a small saucepan and then place it over moderate heat. Keep stirring during the heating process to ensure no clumps for and continue till the sauce thickens. Drop the butter into the sauce and keep on stirring till it melts in.

Then add the lemon juice little by little into the sauce, while whisking it. Then reduce the heat to minimum and add the egg yolk into the sauce. Whisk the mixture till it is smooth and serve it while it is hot.

Creole Frittata | Low Sodium Version

This is a very interesting blend of French cuisine with American cuisine and the flavorsome touch to this frittata makes it a very tasty addition to breakfasts and snacks. This recipe can be doubled but the cooking utensil in use will have to be larger in size. The leftovers from this frittata can be stored in the refrigerator b wrapping tightly.

Preparation Time: 10 minutes

Cooking Time: 15 minutes

Serving: ½ pie serving for 2 people
Sodium per Serving: 456 mg

Ingredients

☐ Spray Olive Oil

☐ Onion (Diced) ½ medium

☐ Eggs   2 large sized

☐ Egg Whites 2 large sized

☐ Water   2 tsp

☐ Salt   1/8 tsp

☐ Fresh Ground Black Pepper

☐ No Salt added Creole or Cajun seasoning blend 1 tsp

☐ Reduced Fat Cheddar Cheese (Shredded) 2 ounces

Directions

Preheat the oven to maximum temperature almost, i.e. 425°F. Then select a small sized skillet r sauté pan and place it over moderate heat. A dash of olive oil will lightly grease the pan. Then fry the diced onions slowly in the pan. The onions should be soft and not very brown but you may caramelize them if you like it that way. Remove the pan from heat.

Mix up the eggs with the egg whites, Creole seasoning (which is available in most markets) and salt and pepper. Whisk this mixture until it becomes frothy.

Put the pan containing the onions back on the heat and pour the egg mixture on top of the onions. Give the pan a good shake to mix well or stir it together. Lower the heat and simmer for around two minutes.

Sprinkle the shredded cheese on top of the whole mixture and pop the pan into the pre-heated oven. Let it cook for around 12 minutes until you can see the frittata puffing up a bit. When you remove from the oven, the texture should not be crumbly but rather firm.

Asparagus Frittata

Asparagus has a nice taste with eggs and this frittata is good for making sandwiches from leftovers. This recipe can be multiplied twice or thrice but a larger cooking utensil will be needed then. If you want to store any leftovers then make sure they are tightly wrapped in plastic wrapper and refrigerated.

Preparation Time: 10 minutes

Cooking Time: 15 minutes

Serving: ½ pie serving for 2 people

Sodium per Serving: 280 mg

Ingredients

☐ Unsalted Butter 1 tsp

☐ Onion ¼ cup

☐ Asparagus Spears 5

☐ Eggs 2 large sized

☐ Egg Whites 2 large sized

☐ Water 2 Tbsp

☐ ParmigianeReggiano cheese 4 Tbsp

☐ Fresh Ground Black Pepper

Directions

Preheat the oven to a high temperature of 400°F. Then place a small to medium sauté pan or skillet and put it on moderate heat. Drop ½ teaspoon of butter into it and let it melt before you add the onions to it. Fry the onions till they become soft and loose the white color. Remove the onions and set them aside.

During the frying, whisk the eggs, egg whites and water together till they become frothy.

Take the asparagus spears and slice their base across to get small rounds. Leave the top two inches of the spears as they are so that they can be used as topping on the frittata.

Slightly increase the heat under the skillet and melt the rest of the butter in it. Add the egg mixture and lower the heat to moderate and let the mixture simmer for around two minutes. After a minute place the asparagus rounds and fried onions into the egg mixture.

Remove from heat and decorate with the asparagus heads and sprinkle the grated parmesan cheese on it as well. Season with freshly ground black pepper. Pop into the preheated oven and reduce the heat down to 350°F. Let it bake for ten to fifteen minutes. The frittata is cooked when it puffs up a bit and gets firm.

Scrambled Eggs With Olives

Preparation Time: 5 minutes

Cooking Time: 10 minutes

Serving: 1 cup eggs for 2 people

Sodium per Serving: 245 mg

Ingredients

☐ Olive Oil 1 tsp

☐ Shallot 1 small

☐ Black Olives (Finely Diced) 6 large

☐ Eggs 3 large

☐ Fresh grounded Black Pepper (To Taste)

☐ Water 1 Tbsp

☐ Parmigiano Reggiano (Grated) 1 Tbsp

Directions

Take a small size skillet and heat it over a moderately high heat. Drop the olive oil in it and let it get hot. Then add the olives and shallot to it and lower the heat. Stir fry them for around three minutes.

During the frying, whisk the eggs and water. Season well with pepper. Pour the eggs over the olives and shallot. After the mixture has cooked for a minute, take a spoon and gently fold the mixture. Keep on doing it until the eggs are cooked. Sprinkle the cheese over it and cook some more and serve right away.

Cereals

Cereals improve digestion and bring a variety of flavors with them. Nowadays cereals are coated with different flavors to be even tastier.

Easy Granola

Combining several cereals with dried fruits and sauces works very well for both adults and kids. Granola is something that is healthy and very interesting to eat. This recipe can be multiplied twice or thrice and is a little time consuming to prepare. But it can be stored at room temperature in a tightly sealed wrap or container for nearly 5 days.

Preparation Time: 15minutes

Cooking Time: 45 minutes

Serving: Single cup serving for 6 people

Sodium per Serving: 39 mg

Ingredients

☐ Water 3 quarts

☐ Steel cut Oats 1 1/3 cups

☐ Quinoa 2/3 cup

☐ Sliced Almonds ¼cup

☐ Chopped Walnuts¼ cup

☐ Unsweetened Applesauce ½ cup

☐ Ground Cinnamon½ tsp

☐ Ground Nutmeg½ tsp

☐ Salt 1/8 tsp

☐ Pure Maple Syrup 2 Tbsp

☐ Raisins ¼ cup

☐ Dried Cranberries ¼ cup

Directions

Preheat the oven to 300°F and place a large saucepan filled with water on high heat. When the water reaches boiling point, add in the quinoa and oats. Once the cereals are added, you can lower the heat and let them simmer for around 12 minutes.

Once they are cooked, drain the water and place under the tap and run cold water on them. Drain them again and put them in a large bowl with the dry fruit, nuts, apple sauce, maple syrup, cinnamon, nutmeg and salt. Fold them together to form a blended mixture

Take a large baking tray and line it with aluminum foil. Spread the mixture onto the tray and pat it down to get a flat surface. Place it in the preheated oven and bake for around 45 minutes. Stir and flatten with a fork after intervals of ten minutes.

Once it is done, remove it and allow it cool completely before consumption and storage.

Healthy Toasted Oatmeal

Oatmeal used to be a staple food for the old English folks and with the passage of time new type rolled oats and quick oats came which could be cooked instantaneously. This recipe is used to make an aromatic version of oatmeal.

Preparation Time: 0 minutes

Cooking Time: 15 minutes

Serving: Single cup serving for 1 person
Sodium per Serving: 246 mg

Ingredients

☐ Quick Oats½ cup

☐ Water½ cup

☐ 2% Milk ½ cup

☐ Salt 1/16 tsp

☐ Light Brown Sugar 1 ½ tsp

☐ Unsalted Butter1 tsp

Directions

Take a medium sized skillet and warm it on moderately high heat. Add the oatmeal to it and cook it for around five minutes. Be sure to keep on stirring frequently or you might get burnt bits of oatmeal. Reduce the heat if you think there is a chance of over-cooking. The toasted oatmeal will look like golden toast and will smell like popcorn.

As soon as the oatmeal is ready, remove it from heat and pour water over it. The water will sizzle at first and

then settle down. This means you can put it back on the stove and reduce the heat to medium heat. Now stir in the milk, sugar and salt till the sugar dissolves.
Keep on cooking it till the liquid has nearly dried up. This will take nearly take five more minutes. When it is done, you can add the unsalted butter and then serve either hot or after it has cooled a bit

Conclusion

Too much salt in your diet is unhealthy. If you want to live longer, you have to reduce your salt consumption. Eat less salt and observe how your health significantly improves. Table salt may be considered a savory condiment but it is a harmful substance you can do well without.

Think of the various diseases you could acquire if you persist with your excessive salt intake. Your heart, kidneys, bones, and your body's homeostasis would all be compromised. Won't it be wonderful to be spending your old age fit as a fiddle, instead of suffering from certain illnesses? It will be disheartening to realize later on that your diseases are caused by your stubbornness to reduce your salt ingestion while you were still young.

This is not saying that you should always eat bland meals. You can utilize the equally savory alternatives listed in chapter 3. You'll satiate your palate and stay healthy at the same time. You've killed two birds with one stone. It's all a matter of perspective and open-mindedness.

Sans other diseases, if you lessen your salt ingestion, you'll no longer feel irritable, or mentally unfocused, and you won't experience muscle weakness unnecessarily. Make a wise choice now and be smart. Limit salt in your diet and live a healthy, happy life.

Part 2

Chapter 1: What Is A Raw Food Diet?

The fundamental principle for the raw food diet is that we should consume plant foods in their natural state. Uncooked and unprocessed foods offer wholesome nutrition for the body. Essentially, a raw food diet is considered a choice towards a healthy lifestyle. It should not be used as a weight loss plan.

It is not easy to stick with a raw food diet, especially when we have indulged in foods that are mostly prepared for us. Devotion to this diet plan requires extensive time spent preparing natural foods. Approximately 75 percent of the diet is fruits and vegetables, which require peeling, chopping, straining and dehydrating the foods for meal preparation.

Staple foods in this diet include:

• Whole grains
• Nuts
• Dried fruits
• Beans
• Sprouted seeds
• Sprouts
• Seaweed

There are four primary categories of raw foodism:

• **Raw vegetarians** – most foods are eaten in their raw state; eggs and dairy are the only animal products in this diet

• **Raw vegans** – most foods are eaten in their raw state; no animal products are in this diet

• **Raw omnivores** – plant-based and animal based foods are eaten raw

• **Raw carnivores** – meat products are consumed in their raw state

Foods Eaten with a Raw Food Diet

Foods eaten in the raw food diet include unprocessed and uncooked items, and omit certain types of foods. Menu selections may vary among raw foodists. Some drink fresh vegetable and fruit juices; others eat foods that have been processed no higher than 115 degrees. The following list represents foods included in this dietary plan.

• Beans
• Legumes
• Nuts and seeds
• Grains
• Fruits and vegetables
• Dried fruits
• Seaweeds
• Sprouts

- Fresh herbs
- Raw spices
- Fresh fruit and vegetable juices
- Coconut milk
- Purified water
- Unprocessed Olives
- Pressed oils
- Raw nut butters
- Vinegars
- Unprocessed raw chocolate (cacao)
- Pure maple syrup
- Raw soy sauce, unpasteurized
- Fermented sauerkraut, miso and kimchee

Chapter 2: Are Raw Food Diets Really Beneficial?

According to raw foodists, foods in their natural state have a vital mix on enzymes that we need. With the right mix, our bodies can digest food fully without using the digestive enzymes in our bodies. Cooking destroys or alters these necessary enzymes, vitamins and minerals. Further, it takes a longer time to digest cooked foods, which can clog our digestive system with fat, carbohydrates and proteins. Raw foods clear our digestive system and also help with detoxification and bloat cleansing.

What are the Health Benefits of a Raw Food Diet?

In addition to the physical benefits, raw foodists also believe there are many health benefits to consuming a raw food diet. Most people who follow this lifestyle report having increased levels of energy, clearer skin and an improvement in losing excess pounds. A raw food diet has low levels of sugar and sodium, and high levels of potassium, vitamin A, fiber, folate and antioxidants.

Increasing these properties in our diet may significantly drop the risk of developing debilitating ailments. Raw foodists are less susceptible to having heart and cardiovascular disease, diabetes, cancer, high blood pressure and high cholesterol.

Typically, raw foods do not have the same amount of Trans and saturated fats found in most cooked foods. This is especially true for processed foods that are prepared for commercial convenience rather than nutritional value.

Not-So Beneficial Side of the Raw Food Diet

The risk of nutritional deficiencies is a primary concern with the raw food diet for most people. A strict raw food diet consists of uncooked, unprocessed plant foods. Not getting enough iron, zinc, vitamin B12 and essential omega-3 fatty acids can pose health risks.

For instance, a vitamin B12 deficiency may cause low HDL and high homocysteine, a building block that develops in the blood stream. Having too little and too much of both respectively increases our risk for heart disease. Multivitamin supplements while following a raw food diet might prevent some deficiencies.

Vitamin B12, a water soluble nutrient, has a vital role in red blood cell production, DNA synthesis and how our brain functions. Consuming a strict vegan diet increases the potential for a deficiency of this nutrient. The only way our body can receive vitamin B12 is from meat, fish and dairy products. Symptoms associated with vitamin B12 deficiency include:

- Fatigue
- Constipation
- Numbness in hands and feet
- Depression
- Memory problems
- Reduced appetite

In addition to supplements, injections or making dietary changes can shift the imbalance.

Restrictions in the raw food diet may also lead to cholesterol problems. Generally, these diets are devoid of fish, peanut butter, cereals and whole grains, which promote positive HDL levels. While we may experience an improvement in triglyceride levels, a raw food diet could hinder the good HDL. An abnormally low HDL increases the risk of heart disease and cholesterol problems.

Poor bone density is another concern for people who follow a raw food diet. Deficiency levels of vitamin D and calcium increases the risk of developing osteoporosis, which is a disease that causes weak and brittle bones that increase risks of fractures. Most raw food diets include low-calorie foods while others may have some calcium. However, not consuming enough leafy greens or vitamin D rich products to absorb the calcium increases the risk of poor bone density.

People with diabetes or hypoglycemia should use caution with this diet plan. While vegetables, fruits and fiber are helpful, an overconsumption of fruit juices could make these conditions worse. Additionally, a raw food diet may not benefit people who have a history with eating disorders because of weight management challenges. Consulting with a health care provider is advised before starting this diet.

Besides the health and nutritional concerns, some people may struggle with staying motivated by this diet plan. Preparation of food requires a tremendous amount of organization. Eating out becomes a challenge since restaurants have very few – if any – raw or partially raw menu selections.

Chapter 3: Potentially Unsafe Foods

The raw food diet offers healthy living techniques for health-conscious people. At the same time, some of the foods consumed in their natural raw state are potentially unsafe. Following is a list of potentially unsafe foods to avoid or consume with caution.

• **Alfalfa sprouts** – contains canavanine, which is a toxin linked to lupus

• Apricot kernels – contains amygdalin, a natural cyanide containing substance

• **Buckwheat** – might be toxic for fair-skinned people when juiced or eaten in large quantities

• **Cassava** – some types, including flour, has toxic properties

• **Kidney beans** – has phytohaemagglutinin, a poison, when eaten uncooked in high concentrations

• **Meat** – harmful parasites, viruses and bacteria are found in raw meats

• **Milk** – subject to Mycobacteria bovis, which can lead to non-pulmonary TB

• **Parsnips** – contains toxic plant-producing furanocoumarins, which acts as a chemical compound against predators

• **Peas** – can lead to neurological weakness in the lower limb

- **Raw eggs** – salmonella bacteria is present in uncooked eggs and may cause serious illnesses.

Chapter 4: What Are Processed Foods?

Generally, consumable products that have been altered from their natural state are considered processed foods. Food manufacturers use various methods either for convenience or safety reasons. The common methods used for processed foods include:

• Freezing

• Canning

• Refrigeration

• Heating

• Boiling

• Sprouting

• Sterilization

Typically, we think that processed foods are bad and do not promote healthy living. However, there are some healthy choices beyond the high-calorie, high-fat snack foods and prepackaged meals. For instance, homogenized milk is pasteurized to kill the bacteria normally found in raw milk. Whereas processed milk defies the principles of the raw food diet, drinking raw milk may cause food-borne illnesses.

Freezing fruits and vegetables preserves natural minerals and vitamins that are essential to our daily health. They are convenient to store and eat year round when frozen. Canned salmon, frozen, unbreaded fish fillets and 100 percent whole grain bread are more examples of processed foods that are good for our daily diet.

As for the bad side of processed foods, we should limit or omit those made from saturated and Trans fats. Large amounts of sugary processed foods can interfere with weight loss efforts. Consuming foods with high sodium content may require bloat cleansing.

Processed Foods That Are Potentially Bad For Our Diet Include:

• Canned foods with high sodium and fat counts

• Frozen dinners and frozen fish sticks with high sodium content

• Refined wheat flour pasta

• Packaged high-calorie chips, candy, cookies and cakes

• Breakfast cereals high in sugar

• Processed meats

In particular, eating processed meats such as bologna, sausage, ham and hot dogs can increase our risk of developing kidney, stomach or colorectal cancer.

Chapter 5: Recipes For Raw Food Meals

Notwithstanding the precautions necessary when preparing raw foods, there are many nutritional values to following a raw food diet. Any method of cooking can alter the nutrient content of most foods, which causes it to lose natural components that our body needs. Vitamin C, folic acid and thiamine lose their nutritional value when foods are cooked. Just sautéing fresh fruits causes a 50 percent decrease in the nutritional value, for example.

We can use pure, unprocessed ingredients in your meals – whether breakfast, lunch or dinner – to create nutritionally dense recipes. Additionally, we never have to sacrifice taste during the transition from traditional recipes.

With raw food meal preparation, we have a greater chance of consuming essential nutrients that our body needs for detoxification and weight management purposes. Raw salads and green sprouts typically contain around 100 calories per pound; fresh fruit has nearly 300 calories per pound. The high water and low fat content make fruits and vegetables low calorie dense foods that can be eaten in larger quantities without adding more pounds. Raw foods with higher calories such as avocado, soaked nuts and starchy vegetables add calories when consumed and help us feel satiated.

With options for buying fresh produce, we can compare prices and the produce offered at different venues. Farmers markets, health food stores and the local grocery stores are ideal shopping places for fresh raw food diet ingredients. As consumers, we can ask for specific items when the grocery store does not carry certain ingredients and a farmers market or health food store is out of reach.

Most raw foodists buy organic and seasonal produce as much as possible for the best meal preparation. Generally, organic foods do not have the pesticides and industrial chemicals found on non-organic foods.

Breakfast

Raw Cinnamon Apple Oatmeal

Prep: 15 minutes

Soak: 24 hours

Yield: 2-3 servings

Ingredients:

1 cup steel cut oats or oat groats

4 medjool dates

2 cups water

1 red apple, chopped

1/2 tsp cinnamon

Pinch of allspice, clove or nutmeg

1 TBS agave nectar, optional

Preparation:

Soak oats overnight in 4 cups of water. Drain and rinse. Soaking the dates make them blender-friendly. Blend oats, dates and water for 25 seconds or until mixture is smooth. Place in a bowl. Mix apples, cinnamon and allspice and add to oats.

Raw Food Breakfast Cereal Muesli

Ingredients:

3/4 cup of raw nuts

Approximately 10 dates, soaked and pitted

2 TBS coconut oil

Fresh mangos, berries or bananas

1 TBS fresh, raw grated coconut

Raw nut milk

Preparation:

Process nuts, dates and coconut oil in a food processor until nuts are finely ground. Add to bowl with fruit and coconut. Add raw nut milk to taste.

Cardamom, Maple And Black Pepper Granola

Yields: 7 cups

Dry Ingredients:

4 cups gluten-free rolled oats
2 cups coarsely chopped raw walnuts

Wet Ingredients:

2 TBS cold-pressed, melted coconut oil
1 oz. raw agave nectar
1/3 cup grade B maple syrup
1 tsp maple extract
1/2 tsp fresh cardamom, ground
1/4 ground cinnamon
1/4 ginger juice or ground ginger
1/4 tsp freshly cracked black pepper
1 tsp sea salt

Preparation:

Soak oats. Drain and rinse until water is clear. Mix oats, walnuts, cardamom, ginger, cinnamon, pepper and salt in a large bowl. In a separate bowl, combine wet ingredients. Pour and stir over dry ingredients until evenly coated.

Place granola on teflex sheet or parchment paper. Mixture will stick to wax paper. Dry for four hours at 105 degrees. Flip batter over and continue drying for an additional 4-6 hours until dry. Break into chunks.

Orange Cinnamon Granola Cereal

Dry Ingredients:

2 cups gluten-free rolled oats

1 cup raisins

1/2 cup hemp seeds

1/4 cup raw sunflower seeds

1/4 cup flax seeds

1/4 cup raw pumpkin seeds

1/2 cup shredded unsweetened coconut

Soak oats, sunflower seeds and pumpkin seeds. Also, dehydrate the oats.

Wet Ingredients:

1/2 cup fresh orange juice

2 TBS orange zest

1/4 cup raw honey or raw agave nectar

3 TBS cold-pressed, melted coconut oil

1 tsp vanilla extract

1 tsp Stevia Powder

1/4 tsp orange extract

1/2 TBS ground cinnamon

1/4 tsp sea salt

Preparation:

Mix dry ingredients in a medium-sized mixing bowl. In a separate bowl, combine and mix wet ingredients. Pour over dry ingredients and stir until well coated. Transfer to dehydrator sheets and dry for 16 to 24 hours at 105 degrees.

Creamy Oatmeal Porridge

Yields: 2 1/2 cups

Ingredients:

1 cup raw, gluten-free rolled oats, soaked overnight
1 1/2 cups water
1 apple, peeled, cored and chopped
2 TBS chia seeds
1 TBS raisins
1 TBS honey or agave
1/2 tsp cinnamon
Dash of salt

Preparation:

Drain and rinse oats until water runs clear. Combine oats, chia seeds, water and raisins in a blender until creamy. Add apple, cinnamon and salt. Continue blending until creamy.

Raw Quinoa Cocoa Pops

Ingredients:

1 cup quinoa grains, sprouted and dehydrated

1 TBS raw cacao powder

2 TBS raw agave nectar

Preparation:

Mix quinoa, cacao powder and agave nectar. Spread into a teflex sheet and dehydrate for 4-8 hours until mixture is crisp and crunchy. Add nut milk to taste.

Peanut Butter Banana Cacao Oatmeal

Yields: 2 servings

Ingredients:

1 cup nut milk
1/2 cup gluten-free oats
2 tsp raw cacao powder
1 TBS chia seeds
2 TBS raw peanut butter
1 ripe, mashed banana
2 TBS raw agave nectar

Preparation:

Combine all ingredients in a bowl and set aside for one hour or overnight. Add favorite toppings such as chopped nuts, strawberries or raisins.

Nutritional Value: 635 calories, 24.6 fat grams, 12.5 grams of fiber, 70 grams of carbohydrates, 20 protein grams.

Raw Autumn Harvest Pumpkin Waffles

Dry Ingredients:

2 cups soaked, sprouted buckwheat

2 cups soaked, dehydrated rolled, gluten-free oats

1 cup soaked and dehydrated raw pecans

1/2 cup dried raisins

1/2 cup shredded coconut

2 tsp pumpkin spice

1 tsp ground cinnamon

1 tsp sea salt

Wet Ingredients:

3/4 cup pumpkin puree

1/2 cup water

1/3 cup maple syrup

1/2 tsp liquid Stevia

Preparation:

Mix buckwheat, oats, pumpkin spice, cinnamon and salt until well coated. Add to food processor until ingredients are in a powdery form. Add wet ingredients and mix until creamy. Transfer to a bowl. Mix pecans, raisins and coconut.

Line waffle iron with plastic wrap and press batter into mold. Cover with more plastic after spreading batter evenly over mold. Close waffle iron and squeeze. Open, remove plastic and lift waffle out, placing it on dehydrator sheets. Dehydrate for one hour; decrease to 105 degrees and continue dehydrating for an additional 16 hours. Remove and serve warm.

Pumpkin Caramel Cereal

Yields: 5 cups

Ingredients:

Dry:
1 1/4 cup raw almond meal

1/4 cup chia seeds

1 TBS pumpkin spice

1/2 tsp sea salt

Wet:
1 ripe banana

1 cup pumpkin puree

1 cup Medjool dates, pitted

1/2 tsp maple flavoring

Hand mix in 2 cups raw, soaked and sprouted buckwheat, 1/2 cup shredded coconut

Preparation:

Pulse together almond meal, chia seeds, pumpkin spice and salt in a food processor. Add wet ingredients. Pour into a mixing bowl and add coconut and buckwheat. Dehydrate on teflex sheets at 110 degrees for 16 hours.

Morning Burst Porridge

Ingredients:

1 cup almond nut milk or purified water

1/3 cup raw rolled oats

1 TBS carob powder

2 TBS chia seeds

1/4 tsp vanilla extract

2 TBS chopped walnuts

1 ripe, chopped banana

Dash of sea salt

Optional toppings: soaked and dehydrated buckwheat, shredded coconut and craisins

Preparation:

Mix all dry ingredients in a bowl. Add remaining ingredients. Mix and refrigerate for one hour or overnight.

Lunch

Easy Vegan Papaya Salad

Ingredients:

2 cups firm green papaya, grated

1/4 cup chopped green beans

1/4 cup grated carrots

1/4 cup cabbage sliced into thin strips

1 TBS soy sauce

8-10 cherry tomatoes, sliced in halves

2 minced garlic cloves

1 small, minced red or green chili pepper

1 tsp lemon or lime juice

1/2 tsp raw sugar (may substitute 1 tsp honey or agave nectar)

1/4 tsp salt

2 TBS roasted peanuts

Lettuce is optional

Preparation:

Combine and toss all ingredients except peanuts. Chill for 2 hours. Add peanuts and serve cold over a bed of lettuce.

Raw Waldorf Salad

Ingredients:

1 cup shredded cabbage

1 grated carrot

1 diced rib of celery

1/2 diced apple

1/3-1/2 cup raw goddess dressing

4 chopped, small dates

Optional - 1/4 cup raw cashes

Preparation:

Toss cabbage, carrot, celery, apple and dressing in bowl. Chill for at least one hour. This softens carrots and cabbage and allows the flavors to mingle. Add dates and cashews, if desired, before serving.

Raw Veggie Chop Salad With Raw Ranch Dressing

Prep: 25 minutes

Yield: 4-6 servings

Ingredients:

1 red bell pepper

1 yellow bell pepper

1 large carrot

1 small zucchini

1 small jicama, or substitute apple

1 green onion, thinly sliced, green part only

Handful sunflower or buckwheat sprouts

2 TBS minced fresh cilantro

Raw Ranch Dressing Ingredients:

1 cup water

1/2 cup macadamia nuts

1 TBS freshly squeezed lemon juice

1 TBS raw apple cider vinegar

1 tsp nama shoyu

1/2 tsp minced garlic

1/4 tsp freshly ground black pepper

Pinch of sea salt, or to taste

Pinch of cayenne, optional

Preparation:

Cut up bell peppers, carrot, zucchini and jicama into thin strips. Place in bowl with green onion, sprouts and cilantro.

Blend dressing ingredients on high speed until they reach a smooth and creamy texture. Allow dressing to chill in the refrigerator for approximately 20 minutes for a thickened consistency.

Toss Vegetables And Enjoy!

Lettuce Wraps

Ingredients:

1/2 cup hemp seed

1/2 cup lemon juice

1/4 cup honey or a few drops of stevia

1 1/2 TBS chopped ginger

1/2 TBS red chili

1 TBS soy sauce

1 cup raw almond butter

1/2 head shredded savoy cabbage

6 very large wild spinach leafs

1 carrot

1 ripe mango

1 handful cilantro leafs

1 handful torn basil leafs

Himalaya sea salt

Preparation:

Cut carrot into small strips. Cut mango into 1/4 inch strips. Puree honey, lemon juice, ginger, red chili and soy sauce in high-speed blender. Add almond butter and blend at low speed. Add water if consistency becomes too thick. Mix almond butter dressing with cabbage in a bowl.

Roll cabbage with dressing into a strip of spinach. Place leaf on a cutting board and add cabbage mix, hemp seeds, carrot sticks, mango, cilantro and basil. Roll up spinach leaf and use a cocktail stick to hold it together. Continue for all spinach leafs until cabbage mix is gone.

Basil And Kale Pesto Salad

Yields: 2 1/2 cups

Ingredients:

1 bunch kale (6 packed cups) stems removed and roughly chopped

2 cups packed spinach

1 cup packed, chopped, fresh basil

1/4 cup extra virgin olive oil

1 clove garlic

2 TBS nutritional yeast

1/2 tsp sea salt

One or two pinches of red pepper flakes

1 TBS raw apple cider vinegar

1/2 cup soaked and dehydrated raw pecans

Salad Makings:

2 zucchini per person, spiralized

Cherry tomatoes, sliced in half

Almond parmesan, for topping

Salt & cracked pepper

Preparation:

Toss cherry tomatoes with zucchini. Set aside. Wash, dry and remove stems from kale. Tear into pieces. Add two cups at a time to food processor with basil and spinach. Break batches of greens down until it spins freely in the processor. Once greens are broken down, add garlic, yeast, salt, red pepper and apple cider vinegar. Mix in food processor. Drizzle olive oil in mixture while processor is running. Stop periodically to scrape down sides. Continue processing until mixture reaches desired texture.

Add pecans and pulse 3-4 times until nuts are broken down and blended into mixture. Coat the noodles and tomatoes with the pesto. Serve with almond parmesan and salt and pepper. Pesto can last in refrigerator for 3-5 days.

Zucchini Noodles With Marinara Sauce

Yields: 4 servings (1/4 cup each)

Ingredients:

1 cup sun-dried tomatoes (soak if hard for 20 minutes)

2 medium ripe tomatoes (seeded and rough chopped)

1 TBS raw agave nectar

1 small garlic clove

2 TBS nutritional yeast

1 TBS cold-pressed olive oil

2 tsp dried oregano

1 tsp balsamic vinegar (or raw apple cider vinegar)

1/2 tsp sea salt

3/4 cup water

4 medium spiralized zucchini

Preparation:

Create spiralized zucchini noodles. Set aside. Combine other ingredients in a high-speed blender. Sauce will be thick.

Nutritional Value Per Serving: 116 calories, 8 grams of fat, 11 grams of carbs, 4 grams of fiber, 1 gram of sugar, 4 grams of protein

Zesty Lime Corn Salad

Ingredients:

4 cups organic corn kernels

1 cup (1 medium) diced red pepper/capsicum

1 cup (1 large) finely diced vine ripened tomato

1 cup (1 large) avocado, diced

1/2 cup (1 small bunch) fresh chopped cilantro

1 TBS (2-3 cloves) finely chopped fresh garlic

2 TBS fresh lime juice

1 TBS cold pressed extra virgin olive oil

1 tsp Celtic sea salt or more to taste

1 tsp cracked black pepper to taste

Preparation:

Soak raw corn in hot water for several minutes. Drain. Combine corn with remaining ingredients.

Nutless Veggie Burger Patties

Ingredients:

1 1/2 cup fresh mushrooms; your choice

1 cup raw sunflower seeds, soaked

Handful of fresh cilantro

1 1/2 cups carrots, rough dice

1/2 cup dried tomatoes

1/4 cup flax meal

1 tsp cumin

1 tsp coriander

1/2 tsp sea salt

1/2 tsp ground chili peppers

Pepper to taste

Preparation:

Mix all ingredients in a food processor. Create patties with a large ice scoop. Place on mesh tray that comes with the dehydrator. Dehydrate for 16 hours or more at 105 degrees. Length of time varies based on how well burgers are done.

Veggie Burger Buns

Ingredients:

2 cups packed, moist almond pulp

1 cup oat flour

1/2 cup Irish moss

1/4 cup date paste

1/4 cup flax meal

3 TBS coconut flour

1 TBS lemon juice

1 Tbsp French Garden Seasoning

1 tsp salt

Preparation:

Make oat flour with raw, gluten-free oats. Blend in a food processor unto flour reaches a fine consistency. Add flax meal, coconut flour, French Garden Seasoning and salt. Pulse until well mixed.

Add almond pulp, Irish moss, date paste and lemon juice. Blend to incorporate all ingredients. May need to add water, one tablespoon at a time, to make dough stick together. Remove batter and shape into buns, approximately 1/4 cup per bun. Roll into balls and flattened with hand.

Place bread on mesh sheet and dehydrate for 6-8 hours at 105 degrees. Touch center to determine if bread is dry enough.

Dinner

Spicy Lemon Pepper Zucchini Pasta With Broccoli

Yield: One serving

Ingredients:

1 medium to large zucchini, spiralized

2 tsp cold pressed olive oil, to start

1 1/2 cups Fresh Broccoli Florets

1/4 cup sliced sun-dried tomatoes (oil packed)

1/2 tsp Hot Red Pepper Flakes

1 tsp Fresh Lemon Juice, or more to taste

1-2 Pinches Sea Salt, or to taste

Black Pepper, to taste

Lemon Zest, for garnish, optional

Preparation:

Create noodles by spiralizing the zucchini. Can use a potato peeler for this step, which leaves a different texture but does not affect the flavor. Sprinkle salt on noodles and allow them to soften. Chop broccoli into smaller pieces. Slice sun-dried tomatoes. Soak in water to soften if not using oil packed sun-dried tomatoes. Combine sun-dried tomatoes, broccoli, red pepper flakes, lemon juice, salt and oil. Toss to coat. Plate and grind fresh black pepper. Add lemon zest if desired.

Chili-Lime Breaded Eggplant

Ingredients:

1 TBS smoked paprika

2 TBS raw apple cider vinegar

3 TBS cold pressed olive oil

1 TBS raw agave, or maple syrup

1 tsp garlic powder

1/2 tsp salt, or to taste

2 TBS water, or a little more to thin mixture

Chili-Lime Chia Seasoning

Eggplant, organic and raw

Preparation:

Peel eggplant and slice. Be careful not to slice too thin otherwise they will become dry and brittle. In a separate bowl, whisk smoked paprika, cider vinegar, olive oil, sweetener, salt and water.

Create a dredging station for eggplant slices, liquid sauce, chili-lime chia seasoning and dehydrator mesh trays. Dip egg plant into liquid sauce, followed by chili-lime seasoning. Coat and shake off excess seasoning. Place on mesh trays to dehydrate at 105 degrees for approximately 10 hours. Length of time depends on desired moistness. Check every 4 hours.

Living Lasagna

Yield: One 7 x 7-inch casserole (4-6 servings)

Almond Ricotta Layers

Ingredients:
1 cup almond cheese
2 TBS raw white miso
1 1/2 TBS red onion, minced
2 tsp nutritional yeast
1/2 tsp crushed garlic
Pinch of nutmeg
Pinch of white pepper

Preparation:

Combine almond cheese, miso, onion, nutritional yeast, garlic, nutmeg and pepper in a medium bowl. Mix well and set aside.

Mushroom Layers

Ingredients:

16 mushrooms, washed and sliced; your choice

1 tsp Tamari or sea salt

2 tsp cold-pressed olive oil

Pinch of pepper

Preparation:

Wash and dry mushrooms, removing all dirt. Do not soak in water. Wipe off with a damp towel. Toss mushrooms in Tamari, olive oil and pepper. Set aside for 10 minutes. Drain and squeeze gently to remove excess liquid.

Noodle Layers

Ingredients:

2 large zucchini, sliced 1/16" thick lengthwise

Sea salt

Preparation:

Place zucchini slices on dehydrator tray, lined with nonstick sheets. Dehydrate for approximately one hour at 105 degrees until soften.

An alternative is to soak for one hour in salt water brine. Drain and towel dry.

Spinach Layer

Ingredients:

1/2 lb spinach, washed and spun dry

Preparation:

Wash spinach leafs and put in a salad spinner to release excess water. Place on dry paper towel and blot dry if you do not have a salad spinner. Place spinach in a food processor until ground without over processing. Squeeze excess moisture from spinach and set aside. Otherwise, puddles of liquid will be in the lasagna.

Marinara Sauce

Ingredients:

6 Roma tomatoes, seeded and chopped (6 cups worth)

1/2 cup sun-dried tomato powder

1 1/2 TBS finely minced onion

1 1/2 tsp crushed garlic

1 1/2 TBS minced fresh basil leaves

1 1/2 TBS minced fresh oregano

1/2 tsp sea salt

Pinch of pepper

Preparation:

You can make tomato powder by dehydrating tomato slices and grinding with a spice/coffee grinder. Scoop out seeds to avoid making the sauce too watery. Place Roma tomatoes in a colander to drain excess liquid. Place in food processor and pulse to chop. The mixture should be slightly chunky like salsa. Add sun-dried tomato powder, onion, garlic, basil, oregano, salt and pepper to processor. Pulse to mix. Let sauce stand for 10 minutes before assembling. This allows the sauce to thicken. Drain off a little juice if sauce is too wet.

Assembly:

Spread layer of marinara sauce in bottom of pan. Place layer of zucchini noodles on top. Next, spread another sauce layer. Add a layer of mushrooms and press with a spatula. Add a thin layer of cheese on top of mushrooms. Follow with a layer of spinach. Press firmly before continuing to layer: sauce, zucchini mushrooms, cheese and spinach. Press each layer firmly.

Serving:

Serve immediately or warm slightly in a dehydrator for 30 minutes to 2 hours at 145 degrees.

Taco "Meat"

Yield: 2 cups

Ingredients:

1 cup raw walnuts, soaked 4-8 hours

1 1/4 cup Portobello mushrooms

1 tsp tamari

2 tsp ground cumin

2 tsp coriander powder

1 tsp garlic powder

1 tsp onion powder

1/4 tsp chili powder

1/8 tsp cayenne powder

Preparation:

After draining and rinsing walnuts, place in a food processor. Add mushrooms, tamari, cumin, coriander, garlic powder, onion powder, chili powder and cayenne powder. Pulse ingredients until crumbly. Be careful not to over blend. To be served immediately or stored in refrigerator for 3-5 days.

Raw Vegan Fish Sticks

Yields: 20 fish sticks

Ingredients:

1 cup soaked raw almonds
1 cup soaked raw sunflower seeds
1/2 cup celery, minced
1/2 cup red onion, minced
1/4 cup fresh lime juice
1 TBS + 1 tsp kelp powder
1 tsp Braggs Aminos or Tamari
1 tsp sea salt
1 tsp dried dill weed, or 1 TBS fresh dill weed
1/2 cup water

Breading Ingredients:
Yields: 1 1/4 cups
1/2 cup raw cashews
1/4 cup ground flax seeds
1 tsp smoked paprika
1 tsp smoked sea salt
1/2 tsp fresh ground black pepper
1 tsp nutritional yeast

Preparation:

Drain and rinse almonds and sunflower seeds. Mix in food processor until they break down to a paste. Add celery, onion, lime juice, kelp powder, Braggs Aminos, salt and dill to processor. Blend, scraping sides down occasionally. Drizzle in water to make the paste moist. Remove and add to a bowl.

Breading Preparation:

Grind cashews in food processor. Be careful not to over process. Add ground flax seeds, paprika, salt, pepper and yeast. Pulse in processor and pour into container for dredging. Measure 2 TBS of batter and shape into a fish stick. Coat stick with breading and place on mesh sheet for dehydration. Continue until all batter is used. Leftovers can be stored in the refrigerator for up to five days. Reheat by placing fish sticks back in dehydrator for a few minutes.

Dehydrate for one hour at 145 degrees; reduce to 115 degrees for 4-6 hours.

Marinated Broccoli And Mushroom Stir Fry

Ingredients:

3 cups mushrooms, sliced

4 cups broccoli, broken in small florets

1 TBS white or black sesame seeds

Cherry tomatoes (add when serving)

Combine in a separate bowl for sauce:

3 TBS olive oil

2 TBS agave nectar

3 TBS Bragg's Liquid Animos or Nama Shoyu

1-2 crushed garlic cloves

1 tsp paprika

1/2 tsp salt

1/2 tsp fresh ground black pepper

Preparation:

Pour sauce over broccoli and mushrooms. Stir well. As vegetables marinate, water is drawn out to create more juice for coating.

You can place bowl in a dehydrator for about one hour at 105 degrees; Allow stir fry to marinate for two hours on countertop; or, marinate in refrigerator overnight.

Quinoa & Goat Cheese Side Dish

Ingredients:

1 cup Quinoa (soaked overnight)
1/2 cup Chopped nuts (your favorite)
1/2 cup Raisins/Craisins
1/4-1/2 cup crumbled, Raw Goat cheese
Pepper, to taste

Preparation:

Mix all ingredients in a bowl and enjoy!

Not Tuna Sandwich

Yield: 3/4 cup (3 servings)

Ingredients:

1/2 cup raw almonds, soaked for 24 hours, rinsed, and drained

1/2 cup raw sunflower seeds, soaked 4-6 hours, rinsed and drained

1/4 cup water, if needed

1/4 cup minced celery

1/4 cup minced red onion

1/4 cup minced fresh parsley

3 TBS fresh lemon juice

1/2 TBS kelp powder

1/2 tsp salt

1/2 tsp dried dill weed or 1/2 TBS fresh dill weed

Preparation:

Run almonds and sunflower seeds through a juicer that has a homogenizing plate. Add small amounts of water while alternating between nuts and seeds. This facilitates the homogenizing process. Put mixture into a large bowl. Add remaining ingredients. Mix well. Serve with a veggie platter, crackers or use as a tortilla filling.

Variations: Add 1/2 cup carrot pulp and dill weed to taste; Put 3/4 cup of Not Tuna on a nori sheet and spread evenly in 1/8 inch layer. Place second nori sheet on top and press, slicing into 12 squares. Dehydrate until crisp at 105 degrees.

Nutritional Value:

274.4 calories; 22.7g fat, 404.7 mg sodium, 13.2g carbs, 5.8g fiber, 2.1g sugar, 9.7g protein

Desserts

Strawberry Rhubarb Cream Cake

Ingredients:

Crust: Yields 3 cups dough

1 1/2 cups soaked and dehydrated raw almonds

3/4 cup shredded coconut

3 TBS raw cacao powder

1/8 tsp sea salt

1 cup organic raisins

1/2 cup prunes

2 TBS water

2+ cups organic fresh strawberries, sliced

Filling: Yields 4 1/2 cups batter

2 1/2 cups rhubarb ice cream mix

1/2 cup organic strawberries

1 cup Rustic Style Rhubarb Sauce

1/2 cup coconut oil, melted

3 Tbsp lecithin, ground or liquid

Preparation:

Crust

Add almonds to food processor and process to a fine crumble. Add coconut, cacao powder and salt. Pulse ingredients together. Add raisins and prunes and process until dough begins to stick together. Rehydrate dried fruit in hot water for 10 minutes if it is too dry. Drain excess water before adding to mixture. Use 2 TBS of water only if batter is too crumbly. Press 2 cups of dough into bottom of pan, pressing firmly and evenly. The remaining 1/2 cup will be used to garnish cake. Cut off green stems from strawberries and slice.

Filing

Melt coconut oil before starting cake recipe. Grind lecithin granules into a powder using a spice or coffee grinder. Combine rhubarb ice cream mix, strawberries and Rustic Style Rhubarb Sauce in blender. Mix until combined. Drizzle coconut oil in blender while mixing ingredients. Add lecithin and continue to blend for another 20-30 seconds.

Pour mixture into pan. Cover and refrigerate for 4-8 hours until cake is firm to touch.

Maple Cheesecake With Cinnamon Swirl Sauce

Ingredients:

Maple Cheesecake Crust

2 cups soaked and dehydrated raw walnuts

1/4 cup + 2 TBS raw agave nectar

2 vanilla beans, scraped (or 2 tsp vanilla extract)

1/2 tsp sea salt

Preparation:

Process walnuts in food processor until mixture become a fine meal. Add remaining ingredients and pulse together. Do not over process nuts because they will release too much oil. Press into pan and set aside.

Maple Cheesecake Filling

3 cups raw cashews, soaked for 2-4 hours

1 1/2 cup raw nut milk

1 cup maple syrup

1/2 cup raw nut cheese

3 TBS fresh lemon juice

2 vanilla beans, scraped or 2 TBS vanilla extract

1/4 tsp sea salt

1 cup raw melted coconut oil

3 TBS lecithin powder

Preparation:

Blend all ingredients except coconut oil and lecithin in a blender for about three minutes. Stop every 44 seconds to test batter. Rub batter between thumb and forefinger to test for grainy feeling. Continue until batter is smooth. Add coconut oil while blender is on. Next, add lecithin, incorporating all ingredients. Pour filling into pan over crust.

Cinnamon Swirl Sauce

1/2 cup maple syrup

1 tsp ground cinnamon

1/4 tsp maple extract

Preparation:

Blend sauce ingredients together until smooth. Transfer to a squeeze bottle with a long tip and small hole. Poke tip of bottle into the batter, squeezing gently. Randomly do this all over cake. Run a toothpick or skewer through areas where sauce was squeezed. Be careful not to disturb crust. Make small dots of sauce on cake surface and run toothpick or skewer through dots to create the swirl effect. Cover with plastic wrap and refrigerate 1-2 hours or overnight.

Chocolate Cherry Chip Bundt Cake

Ingredients:

Outer layer: make 3 batches (2 for walls, 1 for base)
1 cup packed Medjool dates, then soaked for 15 mins.
2 cups almond flour/meal
2 Tbs raw cacao powder
1/4 tsp sea salt

Inner layer:
3 cups Cherry Chip cake batter
2 1/2 TBS raw cacao nibs

Preparation:

Prepare bundt pan with a light coating of coconut oil. Sprinkle a small amount of almond flour inside and tap out excess. Set aside.

Outer Layer Preparation:

Prepare a triple batch of outer layer batter ingredients individually. Use less or more based on pan size. Remove pits form dates and make sure each one is free of bugs or mold. Place in a bowl with hot water. Set aside.

Combine almond flour/meal, cacao powder and salt into a food processor. Pulse together. Darin water from dates and add to mixture in food processor. Continue processing until dough begins to stick together. Dough will create a ball as it spins around.

Dump batter onto wax paper or teflex sheet. Flatten dough to approximately 1/4 inch thick in a circle shape, slightly larger than pan. Life dough carefully and peel teflex off. Lay batter over pan, allowing it to drop in against the sides. Press dough against walls of the pan. Prepare a second batch and use it to piece dough together, creating an even layer up the sides.

Inner Layer Preparation:

Place three cups of the cherry chip cake batter in a medium bowl. Add cacao nibs. Mix with hands.

Assembly:

Pack inside of the bundt pan with the cherry chip batter. Push it firmly and evenly inside pan, stopping approximately 1/4 inch from the top. Make a third batch of the outer dough. Flatten to 1/4 inch thick circle, which should be the circumference of the bundt pan. Remove teflex sheet used to roll out dough and place dough on top of other layers. Smooth and seal cake base.

Let cake chill in refrigerator for a few hours. Place a large plate over the bundt pan to remove the cake. While holding the plate in place, invert pan and plate should drop onto the plate.

Pour ganache frosting over top of cake, allowing it to drizzle down the sides. Top with crushed almonds and cherries if desired. Cake will keep in the refrigerator for 3-4 days when kept in an airtight container.

Snacks

Almond Banana Brittle Cookie Squares

Yields 10 cups batter (72 2×2" squares)

Ingredients:

Wet
2 cups hot water for rehydration
8 oz dried banana, rehydrated in hot water
2 1/2 cups Medjool dates, pitted

Dry

5 cups soaked and dehydrated raw almonds

3 cups coconut flakes

2 1/2 cups soaked and dehydrated rolled, gluten-free oats

1/4 cup flax meal

1 Tbsp ground cinnamon

1 cup of hardening chocolate or vegan chocolate chips

Preparation:

Combine hot water, dried bananas and dates. Soak while preparing remaining recipe. Process almonds in a food processor. Add oats, flax meal and cinnamon. Toss. Place soaked bananas, dates and water into food processor. Blend ingredients until creamy. Pour over dry ingredients. Mix with hands.

Place 5 cups of batter on trays. Spread with hands, pressing down firmly. Score batter into different shapes and sizes. Sprinkle 1/2 cup cacao nibs and pat into batter. Dehydrate for one hour at 145 degrees. Reduce to 115 degrees for an additional 20-24 hours.

Gingerbread Tea Brownies

Ingredients:

2 cup raw hazelnuts

1/4 cup raw cacao powder

1/4 cup dried, unsweetened coconut

6 bags Gingerbread Chai Tea, contents only

1/4 tsp sea salt

1/4 tsp ground cloves

3 cups Medjool dates, pitted

Decorating Options:

Shredded coconut

Dried cranberries

Chocolate chips

Cinnamon Date Frosting

Preparation:

Blend hazelnuts, cacao, coconut, tea bag contents, salt and cloves in a food processor until mixture is finely ground. Add dates, 1/4 cup at a time. Continue processing until well blended. Dough becomes a large ball in food processor bowl. Remove, wrap in plastic wrap and refrigerate 30 minutes or more to chill.

Cover work surface with plastic wrap. Place dough in center and cover with another piece of plastic wrap to prevent dough from sticking to the surface and rolling pin. Roll out dough 1/2 inch thick. Use cookie cutter to cut out desired shapes. Transfer to mesh sheet and dehydrate for 20-24 hours or longer at 115 degrees.

Yummy Chocolate Mint Fudge

Yields: 13 x 9 pan

Ingredients:

2 cups raw soaked walnuts

2 cups raw soaked pecans

1 1/2 cups raw almond or cashew butter

1 1/4 cups extra virgin coconut oil, melted

1 cup raw cacao powder or cacao butter

1 cup raw coconut sugar, powdered in a high-speed blender (very important step)

2 tsp vanilla extract

1 tsp sea salt

1 cup fresh mint, minced

Preparation:

Place soaked walnuts into food processor. Process until nuts are a chunky consistency or finer if preferred. Combine remaining ingredients with the walnuts. Mix thoroughly to fully incorporate ingredients. Line pan with plastic wrap and pour mixture into pan. Press to even out mixture. Set pan in refrigerator or freezer for approximately 30 minutes. Once firm, cut into desired sizes. Keep in refrigerator until ready to serve.

Caramelized Onion Crackers

Yields: 1 tray

Ingredients:

1 cup raw, soaked sunflower seeds

1 cup golden flax seeds, ground

1/4 cup cold pressed olive oil

1/4 cup marinate sauce liquid

3 oz Nama Shoyu or Tamari

2 cups caramelized onions, chopped

Preparation:

Combine sunflower seeds and ground lax seeds in food processor. Pulse until sunflower seeds are broken down in small bits. Add olive oil, marinate sauce and Tamari. Continue processing until well combined. Add caramelized onions and pulse until onions are broken down. Do not turn into paste. Smooth on teflex sheets and score crackers to desired size with a knife or pizza cutter. Place in dehydrator for 8-10 hours at 115 degrees. Turn mixture over and continue drying for an additional 10-12 hours.

"Club" Crackers

Yields 24 – 36 crackers

Dry Ingredients:
1 cup hemp seeds, ground
2 cups almond flour or raw almond flour
1/4 cup natural raw protein powder

Wet Ingredients:
3/4 cup water
2 tsp butter extract
6 drops liquid stevia
Coarse salt for top

Preparation:

Place hemp seeds in food processor and process until seeds begin to break down into smaller pieces. Add almond flour, protein powder and salt. Pulse together. Measure 3/4 cup of water. Add butter extract and stevia to water. Stir together. Pour into food processor and mix into a paste like consistency. Add 1 tablespoon of water at a time if mixture is too dry and clumpy.

Spread mixture on teflex sheet. Dip spatula into water to make it easier to spread. Score crackers into desired sizes. Sprinkle salt on top liberally. Dehydrate for 2 hours at 115 degrees. Remove and make fork markings on crackers. Continue to dehydrate for another 18 hours.

Walnut And Thyme Crackers

Yields: 4 cups of batter

Ingredients:

2 cups zucchini, cubed

1 cups soaked raw walnuts

1 cup soaked raw pecans

1/2 cup golden flax meal

3/4 cup purified water

2 TBS fresh thyme, lightly chopped

2 tsp sea salt

1/2 tsp ground black pepper

Preparation:

You can peel the zucchini or leave the skin on based on your preference. If leaving the skin on, use organic zucchini for the nutrients. If not using organic, peel skin to remove pesticides and wax used to make the zucchini shine. Use dried herbs for the thyme. For flax meal, grind flax seeds in a coffee or spice grinder to a fine powder substance. Transfer into medium sized mixing bowl. Place zucchini into food processor and pulse until vegetable is chopped into small pieces. Keep some texture.

Add zucchini to ground flax. Place walnuts into food processor and pulse until finely ground. Add to flax seed and zucchini mixture and combine. Add remaining ingredients and blend together. Spread 2 cups of batter onto teflex sheet. Score crackers to desired size using a knife or pizza cutter. Dehydrate for approximately 12 hours at 105 degrees. After 4-6 hours, remove teflex sheet and continue drying crackers on mesh sheet for remaining time.

Honey Mustard Pretzels

Ingredients:

2 cups moist almond pulp

2 TBS ground flax seed

3 TBS yellow mustard or raw mustard

1/4 tsp sea salt

1/4 cup almond butter

1 cup almond milk

5 tsp Braggs Aminos or Tamari

3 Tbsp raw honey

1 tsp vanilla extract

Preparation:

Pulse almond pulp, ground flax seed and salt in food processor. Add mustard, almond butter almond milk, Braggs Aminos, honey and vanilla. Process until well combined. Use a piping bag to shape pretzels. Use 1/2 inch for thick and 1/4 inch for thin pretzels. Fill piping bag with batter and work out air bubbles. Squeeze batter out onto teflex sheet. Avoid going too fast, which can cause the line to break.

Sprinkle coarse sea salt or celtic salt on top of each pretzel. Press lightly into dough. Pretzels will not rise since yeast is not one of the ingredients. Dehydrate for one hour at 145 degrees. This sets the outer crust. Cut into 1 inch pieces and place onto mesh sheet. Continue drying for 6-8 hours at 115 degrees. Pretzels will firm up once they cool down.

Tamari Carrot Crackers

Serving size: 1 slice

Ingredients:

4 cups of carrot pulp

1 cup flax-seed, ground

2 TBS tamari

2 tsp turmeric

1 tsp coriander

2 TBS mesquite powder

1 1/2 cup water (as needed)

Preparation:

Place all ingredients in a large mixing bowl. Mix well with fingers, making sure lumps are worked out. Pour batter on two trays on top of teflex sheet. Spread evenly towards edges. Batter will be thick. Score bread sizes and place in dehydrator at 105 degrees or until desired firmness is reached. Store crackers in airtight container for up to four weeks.

Nutritional Value: 92 calories, 4.3g fat, 151.6 mg sodium, 196.9 mg potassium, 10.7g carbs, 6.4g fiber, 2.6g sugar, 3.9g protein

Smoked Paprika Avocado "Fries"

Ingredients:

1/2 cup raw cashews

1/4 cup ground flax seeds

1 tsp smoked paprika

1 tsp smoked sea salt

1/2 tsp fresh ground black pepper

1 tsp nutritional yeast

4 large avocados

Preparation:

Make the breading for these fries by grinding cashews to a small crumb size in the food processor. Do not over process to avoid releasing oils. Add ground flax seeds, paprika, salt, pepper and yeast. Pulse ingredients together and pour into a rectangular container for dredging.

Cut avocados in half, remove skins, slice into 1/4 inch slices and discard seeds. Gently coat avocado slices with the breading mixture and place on the mesh sheet. Dry for 2-4 hours at 115 degrees or until fries are the desired texture. The oil content of the avocado keeps fries from drying crispy.

Chipotle Spiced Sunflower Seeds

Ingredients:

3 cups soaked raw sunflower seeds

3 TBS chili powder

2 TBS olive oil

1 TBS apple cider vinegar

1 clove garlic, minced

1 TBS tamari

1 tsp cumin

1 tsp palm sugar

1/2 tsp salt

1/2 tsp onion powder

1/2 tsp Chipotle

Preparation:

Mix all dry ingredients in a large bowl. Add sunflower seeds and wet ingredients, stirring until seeds are coated. Place in dehydrator for 8 hours at 105 degrees. Store in sealed bag or container at room temperature. Will keep in freezer or refrigerator for months.

Cauliflower Popcorn

Ingredients:

2 heads of cauliflower (sectioned into small florets)
1/4 tsp salt
2 TBS cold pressed olive oil
Nutritional Yeast

Preparation:

Place cauliflower florets in a large bowl and sprinkle with salt. Toss lightly with hands. Drizzle olive oil over top of cauliflower and toss some more with hands. Sprinkle a dose nutritional yeast over top and toss. Add more yeast and toss. Repeat this for about four times, using more yeast. Layer florets on mesh dehydrator screens and dehydrate for 12-16 hours at 105 degrees.

Drinks And Smoothies

Almond Milk

This fresh, homemade recipe is good in smoothies, shakes soups and other raw food dishes.

Ingredients:

1 cup raw almonds

Water for soaking nuts

3 cups water

2 dates (optional)

1/2 tsp vanilla (optional)

Preparation:

Soak almonds overnight in water. Drain water and discard. Blend 3 cups of water, almonds and dates in a blender until almost smooth. Strain mixture using a cheese cloth or other type of strainer. This milk will last in refrigerator up to four days.

Watermelon Limeade Summer Chiller

Prep: 20 minutes

Freezer: 3 hours

Yield: 4 cups

Ingredients:

8 cups seeded watermelon chunks

1/4 cup freshly squeezed lime juice

1/4 tsp vanilla extract, optional

Preparation:

Put half of watermelon chunks in a blender and blend on high for 15 seconds. Pour into ice cube trays. Place in freezer for approximately three hours. Blend remaining watermelon on high for 15 seconds or until desired juice consistency. Add frozen watermelon cubes, lime juice and vanilla. Blend for an additional 10 seconds. Serve at outdoor parties or as an appetizer.

Variations:

You can switch this recipe in many different ways. Add 2 tablespoons of fresh mint leaves, for example.

Raw Chocolate Shake With Raw Cacao

Prep: 10 minutes

Yield: 4 cups

Ingredients:

1 cup raw almonds, walnuts, macadamia or other nuts

4 cups water

4 to 6 medjool dates, to taste

1/4 cup raw cacao powder, or to taste

1/2 vanilla bean, seeds only, or 1 tablespoon vanilla extract

1/4 to 1/2 teaspoon cinnamon, to taste

1/4 to 1/2 teaspoon cardamom, to taste

2 bananas, raw or frozen, optional for thickness

1 TBS raw almond butter, optional for decadence

Preparation:

Blend almonds and water in a blender for 20 seconds at high speed. Pour through a cheesecloth or fine mesh strainer. Rinse blender and pour milk back in. Add remaining ingredients and blend for 20 seconds or until everything is incorporated. Adjust flavors to taste. Best served immediately. If refrigerating until ready to serve, re-blend before consuming.

Purple Kale Green Smoothie

Ingredients:

4-6 kale leaves (use curly or lacinato kale)

1 banana

3/4 cup frozen berries (blueberries, raspberries or strawberries)

1/2 cup water, orange juice or another liquid

1/2 apple, chopped (optional)

3-4 ice cubes

Preparation:

Blend all ingredients in a blender. Add more or less liquid depending on desired consistency for smoothies.

Raw Indian Spiced Chai

This Indian chai tea recipe is caffeine-free, vegan, and suitable for a raw food diet.

Prep: 15 minutes

Soak: 2 hours

Yields: 4 cups

Ingredients:

4 cups water

1 1/2 cups walnuts, almonds or other nuts

4 cinnamon sticks or 1 teaspoon cinnamon

2 TBS green cardamom pods or 1 teaspoon ground cardamom

1/2 tsp whole cloves or 1/4 teaspoon ground cloves

1/4 tsp whole black peppercorns or pinch fresh ground pepper

1/2 cup sliced ginger

1/4 cup agave nectar or to taste

Preparation:

Place all of the ingredients except the agave nectar in a blender and blend on high speed for 30 to 40 seconds or until the nuts are thoroughly ground. Pour the mixture through a fine mesh strainer or cheesecloth. Rinse blender and pour the spiced nut milk back into it. Add the agave nectar and blend for a few seconds. Taste and adjust any of the flavors or sweetener to desired taste before serving.

Avocado Mango Smoothie

Enjoy this gluten-free smoothie as a healthy cholesterol-free vegan breakfast, a nearly raw food breakfast.

Yield: 4 smoothies

Ingredients:

1 fully ripened avocado from Mexico, halved, pitted and peeled
2 cups frozen mango cubes (not thawed)
1 cup orange juice

Preparation:

Combine avocado, mango, juice and 1 cup of water in food processor or blender until smooth. Pour into chilled glasses.

Nutritional value, per serving: 145 calories, 2g of protein, 25g carbs, 4g fiber, 19g sugar, 5g fat, 1g saturated fat

Sweet And Spicy Detox Juice

Yields 3-4 cups

Ingredients:

2 organic apples
3 small red beets
4 cups organic spinach
1 1/2 inches fresh ginger
Liquid stevia to taste

Preparation:

Juicer Method: Place apples, beets, ginger and spinach in juicer. Take a ball of spinach and place it in feeder, followed by the apple or beet to push the spinach through.

Blender Method: Place apples, beets, spinach and ginger into blender. Mix until smooth. Pour mixture through a nut bag. Squeeze juice out in a large bowl. Serve over ice. Compost the pulp or save it for dehydrated crackers.

Juice will oxidize quickly and loses nutritional value, so drink as soon as possible.

Sweet Spinach Hemp Smoothie

Ingredients:

6 cups spinach

2 cups water

3 TBS hemp seeds

1 oz. kale (1 leaf approx.)

5 oz. banana, frozen (1 medium)

3 TBS fresh lemon juice

1 TBS vanilla

1 tsp cinnamon

1 tsp NuStevia Powder

Preparation:

Combine water and greens in a blender at high speed. Add remaining ingredients and blend until smooth. Drink as soon as possible.

Nutritional Value: 375 calories, 14.9 grams fat, 10.6 grams fiber, 51.4 grams carbs, 163.3 grams sodium, 18.9 grams protein

Low Sodium Appetizer:

Crisp potato skins   Serves 2

Low sodium = less than 140 mg per serving

Tip: Get creative with the herbs and spices you use to season the potato skins. Basil, caraway seed, Cayenne pepper, chives, garlic, tarragon, dill and thyme are all great choices.

Ingredients
- ☐   2 medium potatoes
- ☐   cooking spray
- ☐   1 Tbs minced fresh rosemary
- ☐   1/8 tsp black pepper

Directions
1.   Turn oven to 375 F.
2.   Scrub potatoes and prick with knife to vent.
3.   Bake whole potatoes 1 hour or until crisp.
4.   Carefully cut the potatoes in half (use caution: potatoes will be hot)
5.   Scoop out the pulp; allow 1/8" of potato to remain on skin.
6.   Use cooking spray to coat the inside of skin.

7.   Season skins with pepper, rosemary or any seasonings of your choosing.

Bake an additional 5 to 10 minutes then serve.

Nutritional analysis per serving

Serving size: 2 potato skin halves

- ☐   Calories 114
- ☐   Sodium 12 mg
- ☐   Total fat 0 g
- ☐   Total carbohydrate 27 g
- ☐   Saturated fat 0 g
- ☐   Dietary fiber 4 g
- ☐   Monounsaturated fat 0 g
- ☐   Protein 2 g
- ☐   Cholesterol 0 mg

Low Sodium Soup

Soup - Creamy Asparagus Serves 6

Low sodium = 140 mg or less per serving

A great source of vitamin A, vitamin C, folate, iron, magnesium, potassium and selenium. Broccoli can be substituted for asparagus.

Ingredients
- ☐ 2 cups peeled and diced potatoes
- ☐ 1/2 lb. fresh asparagus, cut into 1/4-inch pieces
- ☐ 1/2 cup chopped onion
- ☐ 2 stalks celery, chopped
- ☐ 4 cups water
- ☐ 2 Tbs butter
- ☐ 1/2 cup whole-wheat or whole-meal flour
- ☐ 1 1/2 cups fat-free milk
- ☐ Lemon zest, to taste
- ☐ Cracked black pepper, to taste

Directions

Combine asparagus, celery, potatoes, onions and water in large soup pot. Bring to a boil on high heat. Let boil one minute then reduce the heat and cover. Simmer 15 minutes or until vegetables are tender. Add butter.

Whisk milk and flour together in a small bowl. Add mixture slowly to soup, stirring constantly. Raise the heat to medium high. Stir until soup thickens (5 minutes). Remove from heat and season with lemon zest and cracked black pepper. Serve in warmed bowls.

Nutritional analysis per serving

Serving size: 1 1/2 cups

- ☐ Calories 145
- ☐ Sodium 71 mg
- ☐ Total fat 4 g
- ☐ Total carbohydrate 23 g
- ☐ Saturated fat 2 g
- ☐ Dietary fiber 3 g
- ☐ Monounsaturated fat 2 g
- ☐ Protein 6 g
- ☐ Cholesterol 12 mg

Low Sodium Side Dish

Lemon Rice (with almonds and golden raisins) Serves 4

Low sodium = less than 140 mg per serving

Brown rice has more fiber, vitamins and minerals than white rice.

Ingredients

- ☐ 1/2 cup slivered almonds, chopped
- ☐ 3 Tbsp lemon juice
- ☐ 2 tsp lemon zest
- ☐ 1 cup uncooked brown rice
- ☐ 1 3/4 cup unsalted chicken broth
- ☐ 1/4 cup onions, chopped
- ☐ 1/2 tsp ground cinnamon
- ☐ 1/4 tsp ground nutmeg
- ☐ 1 Tbsp trans-fat-free margarine
- ☐ 1/3 cup water
- ☐ 1/2 cup golden raisins
- ☐ 1 cup frozen peas
- ☐ 2 Tbsp honey

Directions

1. Preheat the oven to 325 F.

2.	Coat baking sheet lightly with cooking spray.

3.	Spread a single layer of almonds on baking sheet

4.	Bake 10 minutes, stirring occasionally, until golden brown.

5.	Remove tray from oven placing almonds on plate to cool.

6.	Use double boiler with water in bottom.

7.	Place the broth, cinnamon, lemon juice, lemon zest, margarine, nutmeg, onion, and rice in top.

8.	Heat, stirring occasionally.

9.	Cover and simmer for 30 minutes (liquid will be absorbed).

10.	In a small saucepan, add the water and raisins. Bring to a simmer, cover and cook for 5 minutes. Add peas and simmer another minute. Add raisin/pea mixture to rice in the double boiler.

11.	Simmer 15 to 20 minutes more (liquid will be absorbed)

12.	Fluff rice mixture and place in serving dish.

13.	Top with toasted almonds and drizzle with honey. Serve immediately.

Nutritional analysis per serving

Serving size: About 2/3 cup

☐	Calories 200

☐	Sodium 66 mg

☐	Total fat 5 g

- ☐ Total carbohydrate 34 g
- ☐ Saturated fat 1 g
- ☐ Dietary fiber 3 g
- ☐ Trans fat 0 g
- ☐ Sugars 4 g
- ☐ Monounsaturated fat 3 g
- ☐ Protein 5 g
- ☐ Cholesterol 0 mg

Low Sodium Main Dish

Yellow Roasted Tomato Sauce over Grilled Chicken   Serves 4

Low sodium = no more than 140 mg of sodium per serving

Grill or broiler is used to cook the chicken and make the smoky-flavored tomato sauce. The yellow tomato sauce also makes this dish unique.

Ingredients
- [ ] 4 yellow tomatoes, halved and seeded
- [ ] 1 1/2 Tbsp extra-virgin olive oil
- [ ] 2 garlic cloves, minced
- [ ] 1 Tbsp balsamic vinegar
- [ ] 3 Tbsp fresh basil, chopped
- [ ] 1/4 tsp salt
- [ ] 1/4 tsp freshly ground black pepper
- [ ] 4 skinless, boneless chicken breast halves, (approximately 5 ounces each)
- [ ] 2 Tbsp fresh flat-leaf (Italian) parsley, chopped
- [ ] 1 Tbsp fresh thyme, chopped

Directions

Prepare charcoal grill, gas grill or broiler. Lightly coat the grill rack or broiler pan with cooking spray (away from heat). Place cooking rack 4 to 6 inches from the heat source.

Arrange tomatoes skin side down on the grill rack or skin side up on a broiler pan lined with aluminum foil. Grill or broil approximately 5 minutes or until the skins begin to blacken. Transfer to a bowl, cover with plastic wrap, and let steam 10 minutes, skins will loosen.

Place olive oil in a small frying pan on medium heat. Add garlic and sauté 1 minute until softened. Remove from the heat and set aside.

Core and peel the tomatoes. Place garlic (with oil) tomatoes and vinegar in a blender or food processor. Pulse until well blended. Stir in 1 Tbsp. of the basil and 1/8 tsp of the pepper.

Sprinkle the chicken breasts with 1/4 teaspoon salt and the remaining 1/8 teaspoon pepper. Stir the parsley, thyme and the remaining 2 tablespoons basil in shallow dish. Dredge the chicken in the herb mixture to coat completely. Grill or broil the chicken until golden brown (about 4 minutes) then turn and brown other side (about 4 minutes).

Place cooked chicken on dinner plates and top with tomato sauce. Serve immediately.

Nutritional analysis per serving

Serving size: 1 piece

- ☐ Calories 235
- ☐ Sodium 287 mg
- ☐ Total fat 7 g Total
- ☐ carbohydrate 8 g
- ☐ Saturated fat 1 g
- ☐ Dietary fiber 2 g
- ☐ Monounsaturated fat 4 g
- ☐ Protein 35 g
- ☐ Cholesterol 82 mg

www.ingramcontent.com/pod-product-compliance
Lightning Source LLC
Chambersburg PA
CBHW062137020426

42335CB00013B/1242